We *CAN* Fix Healthcare
The Future Is NOW

Five Star Reviews
★ ★ ★ ★ ★

"It has been a while since I felt optimistic after reading a book on our health-care system, and yet that best describes my sentiment after finishing Stephen Klasko's new book, *We CAN Fix Healthcare—The Future is NOW*. The book doesn't shy away from all that is wrong with our healthcare system, but the focus is squarely on what can be right about it. If you want to be knowledgeable about the evolution of our healthcare system, and armed with sensible, apolitical solutions, you have come to the right place. Most importantly, this book has been written for the masses, not just the rarified few in the world of health policy. Klasko and crew are tremendously skilled writers who adeptly use humor and self-deprecation to keep you turning the page—while also keeping you hopeful for the future."

SANJAY GUPTA
CHIEF MEDICAL CORRESPONDENT, CNN
PRACTICING NEUROSURGEON

"Dr. Stephen Klasko, the brilliant and visionary CEO of Thomas Jefferson University and Jefferson Health, has written an extremely important and insightful book about how the combination of consumerism and technology can truly transform healthcare from a seemingly hopeless liability of ever rising expenses and shortages into a dynamic industry with more and better care at a lower cost. A mighty wave of breathtaking innovations and breakthroughs awaits us in medicines, medical devices and delivery systems. Klasko and Shea show how all of these dazzling possibilities can become realities . . . and soon!"

STEVE FORBES
CHAIRMAN AND EDITOR IN CHIEF
FORBES MEDIA

"Radical change in business takes a special kind of leadership, and healthcare is no exception. Steve Klasko is such a leader, and his book insightfully explores the transformative process that will finally allow healthcare to join the consumer revolution."

JACK WELCH

FORMER CEO OF GENERAL ELECTRIC AND BESTSELLING AUTHOR

"Cloud, mobility, and big data shifted market power from entrenched incumbent organizations to customers-in-control. Healthcare had missed this message. Dr. Stephen Klasko is a visionary and a courageous healthcare disruptor. As the leader of one of the nation's most forward-thinking medical institutions, he explains in a clear and easy-to-read prose exactly what must be done to transform our outdated healthcare system. Where the politicians and lobbyists failed, the innovators now need to take the lead."

JOHN SCULLEY

FORMER APPLE CEO

"*We CAN Fix Healthcare in America—The Future is NOW*, shows Dr. Stephen Klasko at his best. Merging medical, technical, business and visionary perspectives to drive head-on at challenges and solutions to unwind the Gordian knot of healthcare. Working from the patient perspective inwards, Stephen's approach diagnoses and addresses an exciting and inspiring vision that requires attention."

WILLIAM STEMPER

COMCAST BUSINESS, PRESIDENT

"Dr. Stephen Klasko and Greg Shea travel through time to give us 12 all too logical, innovative, and disruptive prescriptions for transforming healthcare in the universe in which we live. Dr. Klasko can walk the talk, and demonstrates how a systematic and collaborative model can create a healthier system for all."

ROGER HOLSTEIN

CEO, HEALTHGRADES

"We CAN Fix Healthcare—The Future is NOW is a powerful prescription for transcending the grinding inertia and spiraling costs of our healthcare system. With personal interviews of everybody from sick patients to hospital executives—and with an imagined rallying across our otherwise deadlocked political spectrum. Steve Klasko and Greg Shea identify a dozen "disrupters" and offer a compelling fix for one of our country's most vital but also most obstinate institutions."

MICHAEL USEEM
PROFESSOR OF MANAGEMENT AND
DIRECTOR OF THE WHARTON LEADERSHIP CENTER
UNIVERSITY OF PENNSYLVANIA

"What a reprise! Klasko and Shea have done it again with the right mix of wisdom, straight fun, and well intentioned satire. Now if only the policy makers would listen up."

ELLIOT SUSSMAN, MD
CEO, THE VILLAGES HEALTH

"This book about the future of healthcare in the United States is surreal, but certainly no more surreal than the current reality we all experience. The authors take us through a time-travel enabled vision of a new "impossible" future for American healthcare and the health of America. The trip is light-hearted, even joyful, but simultaneously it is intensely serious. We are invited to "look in the mirror" for "impossible" solutions for current healthcare conundrums— solutions that simply appear to be common sense when looked at from afar. This book will make you smile as you bounce through its kaleidoscopic scope. But, more importantly, it will make you think. Hopefully, it will also make you, whoever you are, act. Read it for fun, but beware the "vapors." You may never see the world of healthcare in the same way again."

ROBERT J. LASKOWSKI, MD, MBA, FACP
SENIOR FELLOW, SCHOOL OF PUBLIC POLICY, UNIVERSITY OF DELAWARE
PRESIDENT AND CEO (RETIRED),
CHRISTIANA CARE HEALTH SYSTEM, DELAWARE
CHAIR, BOARD OF DIRECTORS,
ASSOCIATION OF AMERICAN MEDICAL COLLEGES

"Whether you're a healthcare professional, policy maker, healthcare entrepreneur or technologist, this book will compel you to take action. Stephen Klasko challenges us, inspires us, and puts us squarely on the path we must take to change, innovate and bring about a healthcare system that works for everyone."

JOHN DOERR
KLEINER PERKINS CAUFIELD & BYERS

"The crisis in healthcare isn't political, it's a crisis of leadership. Steve Klasko is saying step up! Make change an opportunity to lead, not follow. And he shows exactly how. I love his argument that every so called disruption can be transformation if we seize the moment and lead. This book is telling us to lead the future, don't be afraid of it, and make America [have] the best healthcare system anywhere, for everyone."

JUDITH VONSELDENECK
PRESIDENT AND CEO, DIVERSIFIED SEARCH, INC.

"This book is a must read for anyone who cares about the future of healthcare in America. It makes the case that to improve our healthcare system we must disrupt almost every element of our current system. It is a fascinating and electric first person narrative that often makes me laugh but always made me think!"

EDWARD RENDELL
FORMER GOVERNOR OF PENNSYLVANIA AND
CHAIRMAN, DEMOCRATIC NATIONAL COMMITTEE

"Stephen Klasko and Gregory Shea are gadflies with bona fides—disruptors with a plan. With visionary insight and a light touch, Klasko and Shea offer *We CAN Fix Healthcare—The Future is NOW* as a crucial dispatch from the future frontlines of medicine and a clarion call to revolutionize the American healthcare system as we know it."

AJAY RAJU
DILWORTH PAXSON LLP

We *CAN* Fix Healthcare

The Future is NOW

Stephen K. Klasko, MD, MBA

Gregory P. Shea, PhD

with Michael J. Hoad, MA

Mary Ann Liebert, Inc. publishers

Library of Congress Cataloging-in-Publication Data

Names: Klasko, Stephen K., author. | Shea, Gregory P., author. | Hoad,
  Michael, author.
Title: We can fix healthcare in America : the future is now : decision 2016 /
  Stephen K. Klasko, Gregory P. Shea with Michael Hoad.
Description: New Rochelle, NY : Mary Ann Liebert, Inc. Publishers, [2016] |
  Includes bibliographical references and index.
Identifiers: LCCN 2016013815 | ISBN 9781934854426 (pbk. : alk. paper)
Subjects: | MESH: Health Care Reform | United States
Classification: LCC RA445 | NLM WA 540 AA1 | DDC 362.10973—dc23
  LC record available at http://lccn.loc.gov/2016013815

ISBN: 978-1-934854-42-6
ISBN (e-book): 978-934854-43-3

Mary Ann Liebert, Inc.
140 Huguenot Street
New Rochelle, NY 10801

To Lynne, David, and Jill
for not allowing me to take myself too seriously

To Colleen
for making sure that I take some things seriously

— STEVE KLASKO —

To Iris
for everything

To Emelyn and Meredith
for continuing to share the vistas that are their lives.

— GREG SHEA —

To Caroline and Lillian
with great love

— MICHAEL HOAD —

Contents

"You never change things by fighting the existing reality. To change something, build a new model that makes the existing model obsolete."

— R. BUCKMINSTER FULLER —

"I attribute my success to this . . . I never gave or took any excuses."

— FLORENCE NIGHTINGALE —

"Impossible is just a big word thrown around by small men (and women) who find it easier to live in the world they've been given than to explore the power they have to change it. Impossible is not a fact. It's an opinion. Impossible is not a declaration. It's a dare. Impossible is potential. Impossible is temporary. Impossible is nothing!"

— ADIDAS MARKETING CAMPAIGN —

"Everyone's got a plan . . . until they get punched in the mouth."

— MICHAEL TYSON —

"Do or do not. There is no try."

— YODA —

Contributors

Praveen Chopra

Anne Docimo, MD

John Ekarius

Neil Gomes, MMS, MEd

Bruce Gresh, PhD

Nicole Johnson, DrPH

Jack J. Kelly, MD

Sidney and Caroline Kimmel

Bernie Marcus

Daniel A. Monti, MD, MBA

Donna Petersen, ScD

Alexandra Printz (MD 2016)

Lauren Ashley Sharan (MD 2016)

Gregory Snyder, MD

Roderick Thompson (MD 2016)

Navin Vij, MD

Jack and Suzy Welch

Andrew Young

George Zabrecky, DC, MD

Acknowledgments

We gratefully acknowledge the more than 100 individuals from all walks of healthcare who were interviewed for this book. The book is written as a first-person narrative by **Steve Klasko,** but it reflects a huge number of viewpoints, considered opinions, and expert thinking.

The quotations in this book are real—exact quotes or close paraphrases. A more in-depth look at the raw interviews is highlighted under the "Interviews Unplugged" section after the narrative.

Joined by a group of medical students, we asked a standard set of questions of people who are patients and families, advocates and activists, professionals and clinicians, leaders and experts, even academics. You'll see in the quotations that we asked for the good and the bad of healthcare today. And then we asked them to consider an ideal healthcare system constructed without blaming one group or another.

For us, this is the core thought experiment: If we can imagine an ideal healthcare system of the future, what can we do today to make that happen? This book contains many of the answers we got from all those we asked.

We are not the experts. They are. You are. Now we all have to make

. . . the future happen, together.

Preface

Healthcare needs a "new model" that makes the existing failed model obsolete. Obamacare, accountable care organizations, and bundled payments are all part of the new strategy, but as we enter the next fifteen years of the twenty-first century, we are still getting "punched in the mouth" with rising costs, rising health disparities, and anger on both sides of the aisle. Yet, we are still told that it is "impossible" to fundamentally transform our complex, inefficient, expensive, inequitable, and occasionally unsafe healthcare delivery system. Everyone—physicians, patients, pharmaceutical companies, employers, payers, policy makers, academic leaders, administrators, information technology vendors—says, "I'm trying to fix it. It's not me it's them!"

So, why another book on healthcare in America? Bookshelves and search engines overflow with them. The topic matters to us individually and collectively, but why add to the pile? Actually, we think this book differs from most of the pile in several notable and, we would argue, useful ways.

First, **we don't presume that we are the smartest people in the room.** We think that we are more than smart enough and experienced enough to make a contribution at an important time, but we don't think or write—either explicitly or implicitly—as if everyone else should just shut up, sit down, and do what we say. We don't think others need only to follow us to find healthcare nirvana, nor are we angry that they haven't. We think we have something to say that could help, and yet we don't take ourselves too seriously to play a bit in the process of saying it—a spoon full of sugar and all that. This stance on our part, we believe, allows a broader, fuller look at healthcare in America and a more enjoyable read.

Second, **we firmly believe that the key word in the phrase "the system of healthcare in America" is the word *system*.** Our country has evolved an overall approach to healthcare in this country. We've built it over time, and while it's not pretty to look at in its entirety, in its "system-ness," it all fits together. Our system of healthcare, like any system, delivers what it is designed to deliver. Hence, to produce something else, something such as better outcomes and better care for less cost, for instance, requires stepping back and looking at the system as a whole. To change a part and thereby to expect system change probably stems from either naiveté or cynicism. In either case, failure to address the whole leads to changing only a part (which produces minimal, if any, change in the whole.) We look at the system as a whole in this book. We then use that lens when considering the component parts and their interconnection. That perspective makes this book different as well.

Even *looking* at the whole, let alone *changing* it, has proved frustrating and repeatedly difficult. It's easier to try to fix pieces. Looking at the healthcare system as a whole inevitably triggers opposition. Yet, how one *looks* serves to determine how one *sees* (to paraphrase **R. D. Laing**, Scottish psychiatrist and author) and how one *sees* determines how one *acts*. In the case of change, the way of looking at it models the change you get.

If one wants to change the healthcare system in America, then three things need to happen:

The values behind this book:

1. We need to **objectively examine the whole system**. As a physician you would not treat a patient based on indirect examination, innuendo, or a sense of inevitable failure.

2. We need to **look in the mirror**. It is way too easy to absolve yourself no matter what your role in the system, whether Democrat or Republican, provider or patient, employer or insurer. You own it, its successes and its failures.

3. **Do or do not. Yoda** had it right. As we approach yet another election cycle, it is time to decide that we are willing to fundamentally disrupt the system or resign ourselves to what we have. Incremental "mission accomplished" changes just serve to move the blade in the wound, prolonging the agony.

President Obama provided painful confirmation of the previous paragraph. His campaign included a pledge that he would redesign America's healthcare system by putting the key stakeholders, representatives of all of them, in a room and have them work through the matter on C-SPAN for all to see.

Brilliant.

Lay out (expose?) the system to one and all and, in so doing, educate all of us as policy makers, providers, and patients embed a system-wide approach to system-wide change.

Brilliant.

One problem. It didn't happen. Doors closed. Side deals and sub-optimization reigned yet again. Lots of froth and frenzy begot, thus far, minimal change in desired outcomes such as actual, aggregate, affordable access to improved healthcare. The process augured the result. Hence, the authors seek to go back to what President Obama did not do in order to go forward. What if he had assembled those stakeholders? What if he did it before he left office? What if his successor chose to go back to go forward? Doing so would have differentiated Obamacare and does differentiate this book.

Third, **we remain optimistic.** We wrote *The Phantom Stethoscope: A Field Manual for Finding an Optimistic Future in Medicine** in order to identify challenges facing physicians who wished to shape the future of medicine and to support them in that work. We have had the exceptional opportunity over the intervening decade and a half to work with physicians and other healthcare providers, along with many other healthcare stakeholders, to do just that. That work and those people have improved healthcare outcomes and lowered its cost to the great satisfaction of patients and providers alike. We know, therefore, that people can make healthcare fundamentally better, and not just in a moment—however important a moment might be—but over time. We have seen it. Time and time again.

America has all the ingredients necessary to provide better, cheaper healthcare. It needs chefs who are willing to do, not just try.

---

* Stephen K. Klasko, and Gregory P. Shea, *The Phantom Stethoscope: A Field Manual for Finding an Optimistic Future in Medicine*, Hillsboro Press, 1999.

The authors combined have taught healthcare, presided over health systems, taught around the world, seen successes and failures, started healthcare companies, and been patients. That experience gives us the ability and, we daresay, the right to offer considerations for the national discourse. We do not offer jeremiads. We offer focus and energy based on optimism born of experience and a view of what could be. That perspective differentiates this book as well.

As part of the research for this book, we interviewed dozens of healthcare stakeholders—patients, providers, insurers, employers, health policy makers, information technology specialists, healthcare chief executive officers, administrators, entrepreneurs, regulators. You name them—if they are involved in healthcare (who isn't?), we interviewed them.

We asked them several questions that form the foundation for this book.

1. If you could wave a magic wand, what are three things you would like to say about healthcare in America that you cannot say today?

2. That said, then what's most wrong with America's healthcare system today?

3. What do you believe people most need to understand in order to better get a grasp of your world, of your part of the healthcare system?

4. Which stakeholders/players are the biggest impediments to fixing America's healthcare system? What's the one thing they could change to most improve healthcare in America?

5. What might other stakeholders say is your biggest contribution to what's wrong with healthcare in America? What's the one thing that you could do differently that would most positively impact healthcare in America? Why don't/can't you do it?

This is the second book after *Phantom Stethoscope* in which the authors have utilized a history of the future approach. These techniques free the author and the reader of current noncreative constraints. They also rest upon the assumption that an alternative and desired future can exist and that one can achieve them. The techniques then advocate working backward to connect the future to the present while, again, assuming success. History of the future advocates "begin with the end in mind." Backcasting guides planners through a disciplined step-by-step backward walk from the future to the present. Working with scenes takes planners from the future to consideration of the organizational redesign necessary to yield that desired future to the changes required to produce that design.

It's also a lot more fun to write and hopefully to read. These techniques can transport a reader to another vantage point, to one freer of limits, filters, and biases of our current moment. Such transportation can free the mind to consider new possibilities or options. It can also lead to discovery of an energy source for change: excitement born of envisioning a better world.

So, to quote Yoda* again. "Difficult to see. Always in motion is the future."

In that vein, may the *fours* be with you.

1. Affordable, accessible healthcare regardless of race, religion, or preexisting conditions.
2. Training the providers of the future, not the past.
3. Allowing healthcare to join the consumer revolution.
4. Aligning incentives and creative partnerships between patients and providers based on improvement of health individually and collectively.

Here's to realizing an optimistic future in American healthcare for all of us, our children, and their children!

---

*Yoda (from Wookiepedia): one of the most renowned and powerful Jedi Masters in galactic history. Standing at about 66 cm tall, he was a male member of a mysterious species. First seen in 1980's *Star Wars* epic, *The Empire Strikes Back*.

How It All Came to Pass

PHILADELPHIA, PA, 2026: Time to recall how we—all of us—with a little help from patients, pop culture, and **Harry Truman**, transformed healthcare in America. No one thought it could be done. Tonight, I'm writing this up for *Healthcare Transformation* (www.HTboldhealth.com), the journal that helped us talk to each other as we built the completely new world of care that we see today.

As **President Obama** tells it, he was alone with his thoughts at last in the Oval Office . . . gun control, climate change, wars, peace, and oh yeah, healthcare reform. The hard work of bending the arc of history. What else could he affect in one last year?

And then **Harry Truman** walked in.

No "hello." No "how did you get in here?" Truman was direct. "Assemble a national healthcare conference."

I'm sure President Obama's first thought was obvious: "Well, this is what happens when you live in the White House—hallucinations about other guys who lived here. Now Truman. And a conference?" "Now *that*'s strange and pointless!" he said out loud in a patient, if marginally patronizing, voice, "Why would I want to call yet another gathering on healthcare?"

The man from Missouri drew a bead on the president and said, "Because it's important business that remains unfinished, for you and for me. Let me tell you what I said seventy years ago. And, yes, don't tell me you solved it. We both made a start. We both have to finish it."

President Obama glanced at the heading of the typed (typed!) papers.

Special Message to the Congress Recommending
a Comprehensive Health Program

Harry S. Truman*   November 19, 1945

"You really are Harry Truman?"

"That buck stops here" the man responded, and the president leaned
back in his chair.

"But I was a man in shock when I reviewed our healthcare in 1945.
More people were dying of illness every year than we lost in the entire
war. Worse: You think of older people as sick. But what we learned in
the war was that 30 percent of young men and women were rejected
from conscription because of physical or mental incapacity. We were
rejecting 47 percent of Americans in their thirties. You and I must resolve that no child come to adulthood with diseases or deficits that
could be addressed in childhood. And even worse: We saw that the poor
have more sickness but less care.

"I'm telling you, 'No people have ever done more than Americans
to understand how to treat maladies while doing so little to secure wellness and well-being. That must and can change.'"

President Obama gazed downward more than a bit dejectedly. "I
and many others have tried."

Truman leaned over the desk and said, "Then try again, but try differently. America was not built on fear. America was built on courage, on
imagination and an unbeatable determination to do the job at hand."†

"OK, could you be more specific?"

Truman then offered, "Think patients. Just like you thought about
your mother and her illness. It's personal. Think systems. It's the
whole thing, not the pieces. Remember that systems give you what they
are designed to give you. Get the whole damn thing in one room. And
make the whole thing transparent. You got that right and then backed
down. Don't do that again."

---

* A full copy of this concise and uncomfortably current speech appears in the "Special
Message" at the end of the book.

† Indicates actual HST quotes.

Silence. Hard looks between powerful entities.

President Obama leaned forward, "And if for some strange reason I decide to call this conference and cash in my chits to get representatives of America's healthcare system there, then you will do the rest?"

"Yes."

"How?"

"Leave that to me," he said, "along with some pretty unusual colleagues from many realities. Think of them as the ark of history to help you with the arc of history."

"Deal."

President Obama and President Truman shook hands.

"You know the hard part?" President Obama said. "Since your era, this country has split in two over almost ever issue. It's not about facts. It's about ideologies. I am very worried."

"You should worry. Remember what **Benjamin Franklin** said when asked upon exiting the U.S. Constitutional Convention in 1787, 'What have we got—a Republic or a Monarchy?'" He responded, 'A Republic, if you can keep it.' Just like in healthcare. It's up to us.

"But remember what I said: Keep it personal for patients. Fix the big system. And make sure everything is transparent, from what you're doing to every blasted hospital bill every patient gets."

Truman disappeared. Obama looked at his daily calendar and muttered, "I've just *got* to get a new chief of staff."

As for what happened at the conference? Well, that's what this book is about. So, please, read on for the first first-person account of the last healthcare conference we'll ever need.

CHAPTER 1

When Politics and Healthcare Became Fun Again

In 2026, Steve Klasko looks back on THE EVENT—the great change that finally transformed healthcare*

2016.

The year we all came together. The Summer of Love† sequel.

2016 was the presidential campaign, now viewed as the *least* divisive related to healthcare in several decades. The presidential health platforms were remarkably similar in their aspirations, albeit with slight differences in the role of government and sources of revenue. (After all, there had to be some reason for cable news to exist.)

2016 was the year we decided that all the stakeholders could get together and actually create a new model of healthcare based on solutions to decades-old problems that united the payers (employers, government, and patients) with insurers and providers. And included everyone else in the complex healthcare ecosystem.

No, I'm not on drugs.

I'm not crazy.

This is not science fiction (although how it came about certainly was).

It is real.

---

* "I" refers to our chief memorialist, Steve Klasko.

† Summer of Love: refers to a social phenomenon that occurred in 1967 when, through a strange series of events, young people gathered together toward a brighter future. Summer of Love 2016 refers to the strange series of events that led to the Democrats and Republicans getting together toward a brighter healthcare future.

Within the last few days, the Republican party and Democratic party published their healthcare platforms, and they are remarkably, eerily, excitingly similar and optimistic.

The Democratic platform is aptly named *The Dramatically Different Democratic Discourse on a New Healthcare for America (DDDD)*.

And in this corner, the Republican platform is equally aptly named *Let's Re-imagine a Republican Revolution in Healthcare, Rather Than Repeal (RRRRR)*.

Don't believe me? Here they are. Side-by-side. Direct quotes are included. What's remarkable is the total agreement on the twelve principles.

1. **Look at healthcare as a team sport and develop a system that is both user-friendly and delivers value.**

DDDD	RRRRR
"The federal government will reduce Medicaid/Care funding to states that refuse to allow nurse practitioners, midwives, pharmacists, and other clinicians to practice at the highest level of their degree and licensure."	"The federal government will begin a massive review to remove federal regulations that unnecessarily limit scope of practice by physicians and licensed health-care providers to achieve the best care for their patients."

2. **Take the volume incentive out of the payment system and put incentives in place that are aligned with optimal health outcomes.**

DDDD	RRRRR
"The federal government will accelerate the shift of paying for fee-for-service to paying for value to a population. Our goal is to keep people well and prevent expensive and difficult care."	"The federal government will work with private insurers to create incentives for good health, exercise, and diet—core components of a healthy lifestyle."

3. **Provide the right solution for the right patient at the right time and provide coordinated care across patient condition, services, and time.**

DDDD	RRRRR
"The federal government will accelerate funding for precision medicine and data analysis to ensure legally defensible personalized care for each patient."	"The federal government will work with private insurers, health systems, and doctors to reform malpractice legislation and provide tools for appropriate care, not defensive care."

4. **Select and educate physicians of the future as opposed to those of the past. Thou shalt never again be surprised that doctors (solely based on science GPA, multiple-choice tests, and memorizing organic chemistry formulas) are not more empathetic, communicative, and creative.**

DDDD	RRRRR
"The Department of Education will work with accrediting bodies to speed the selection and licensing of physicians using criteria of communication skills, behavioral and social knowledge, and facility with using data analysis to provide personalized care for patients."	"We will match America's world-leading high technology with the humanistic, trusted tradition of doctors, nurses, and health teams to help patients understand and plan their lives to be well, to overcome illness, and to be comforted at the end."

5. **Use technology to ensure that every surgeon can objectively prove appropriate competence and confidence to perform the requested procedure.**

DDDD	RRRRR
"By 2018, the DHHS and other governmental agencies will establish metrics of technical and teamwork competence and models and measures such that every patient knows their doctor has proficiency in the procedure performed."	"By 2018, specialty societies will establish metrics of technical and teamwork competence and models and measures such that every patient knows their doctor has proficiency in the procedure performed."

6. **Learn the lessons of the now-defunct Blockbuster and move healthcare from a "come to my hospital when you are sick" to a Netflix mindset of "getting healthcare out to where**

the consumer is." **Do not build new inpatient beds when it is clear that there will be disruptive influences that fundamentally decrease the need for expensive inpatient beds.**

DDDD	RRRRR
"The federal government will incentivize the infrastructure for personalized care in any location, reducing barriers to tele-health and forcing interoperability of electronic health records."	"We will work with private industry to reduce the burden of the computer in the doctor's office, providing new tools for physicians and their teams to guide patients through their lives."

7. **Always send a patient a believable, understandable bill for services rendered in a manner that clearly states what was done, what it cost, and what the patient owes—regardless of who is paying the bill.**

DDDD	RRRRR
"The federal government will require transparent billing to patients, including cost estimates in advance, especially at the end of life."	"The government will work with doctors, health systems, and insurers to ensure that patients will not be bankrupted by care and can be guided through decisions about costs of treatment, especially at the end of life."

8. **Never use the term "alternate healthcare" for modalities used to treat chronic diseases that are utilized by patients and providers in other countries, and in some cases, have much better results than traditional American medicine in treating said diseases.**

DDDD	RRRRR
"DHHS and other governmental agencies will mandate and provide funding for any patient with a chronic disease that chooses to explore non-traditional therapy or therapy predominately utilized in other countries."	"The government will create tax incentives for healthcare companies or providers that develop outposts such that patients with chronic diseases will have more options outside of traditional American medicine."

9. **De-fragment the application of innovation and clinical research through super-sites. Thou shalt cease and desist constructing walls between institutions of non-interoperability that hamper the acceleration of research and innovation.**

DDDD	RRRRR
"The government will create a 'New Deal' for innovation, with stimulus funding for cooperative partnerships between universities, between universities and cities, between universities and private industry."	"Congress will remove all barriers to innovation, holding all entities that receive government funding accountable for ensuring America's role as the world leader in patents, entrepreneurship, and cures for intractable disease."

10. **Create an integrated, interoperable, legacy electronic health record system allowing for vendor-driven, patient-centric apps such that your health information is at least as integrated as your shopping information on AMAZON or your viewing information on NETFLIX.**

DDDD	RRRRR
"Government shall develop (with the help of the private sector) a single, interoperable health record that is owned by the patient and able to be shared across healthcare venues."	"The private sector shall develop (with the help of the government) a single interoperable health record that is owned by the patient and able to be shared across healthcare venues."

11. **Understand systems thinking and employ said models in your attempts to redesign a healthcare system that actually makes patients and communities healthier. Only then will you be able to "break" the iron triangle of access, quality, and cost.**

DDDD	RRRRR
"The federal government will create incentives for America's healthcare leaders, payors, and innovators to pioneer models of private and public funding for all Americans."	"We will work with America's innovators and healthcare leaders to protect this nation's world-leading, highest quality healthcare and to pioneer business models that provide that care to those less fortunate."

12. **Never again be satisfied with *any* healthcare disparities based on race, creed, religion, sexual orientation, socioeconomic status, or planet of origin.**

DDDD	RRRRR
"The federal government will create a "disparity scale" to accompany its satisfaction scales in rating health plans and providers. We will work to make the 'patient bill of rights' extend to the system of providing care without disparities."	"We will build incentives and remove regulations to encourage the ideas that make 'healthcare for all' good business. America is founded on the idea that all of us are created equal, and that principle applies to healthcare."

If you are reading this book before Election Day 2016, this is how it will happen—you can bank on it. If you are reading this book after the election of 2016, you already know about how we came together around healthcare transformation, the boon to the economy, and the parties and jubilation around this optimistic healthcare future.

If, for any reason, that is not the world you are living in, then you are in an alternate universe* to mine because I have been there and back, and believe me, this is just what happens.

"So," you might ask, "If that's the case, why go any further? Who's going to buy this book if all the answers are in Chapter 1?"

First of all, I might argue, you already bought the book. Or you are reading the excerpt from this book in our journal *Healthcare Transformation.*† Or you are doing something illegal that has gotten you to this chapter without paying, in which case it would be great to have your email address.

But the main reason is that, while we have told you *what* happened, nobody (until now) knew how it happened.

Those twelve principles that everyone so easily embraced—what have euphemistically been called the **"Twelve Disruptors of the Demise of the Old Healthcare"**? How did they get to us, and how did everyone agree?

---

* Alternate universe: a separate, self-contained reality existing with our own.

† *Healthcare Transformation:* a peer-reviewed journal committed to exploring new and better models to deliver and teach healthcare, published by Liebert Publishing.

That is the story and that is why you should continue reading to Chapter 2 and beyond.

I promise you it's fun, you'll learn some stuff you didn't know before, and, most importantly, you will understand the "behind-the-scenes" story of how all of us decided to, as the Youngbloods* sang in the first Summer of Love, on behalf of healthcare in America, "Get together, learn to love one another right now . . . right now . . . right now!"

---

* The Youngbloods: an underappreciated 1960s rock group whose major hit, "Get To-gether," was the "national anthem" for the Woodstock generation.

CHAPTER 2

My Trip There and Back *or* I Was There When Healthcare Was Reinvented

It's been ten years already!" That was my first reaction when I was asked to attend the anniversary celebration of what is now viewed as the "breakthrough moment" for the new healthcare back in January 2016. As with any momentous event, you always try to relive your thoughts and emotions back when it happened. I'd love to say that we all knew that this meeting would be a turning point in transforming the fragmented, consumer-unfriendly healthcare in America of the early 2000s and 2010s to the bastion of social, economic, and technologic envy of most of the rest of the world. But we didn't. In fact, when I first got the notice asking me to attend an invitation-only summit in Big Sky, Montana, my reaction was more of a virtual eye roll than any anticipation that I would be witnessing history in the making.

Not that the thought of traveling to the mountains for a week and leaving the daily grind and stress of leading an academic medical center was a sacrifice, but in the context of 2016, the chances of anything worthwhile coming out of this was equivalent to the odds that my beloved PHILADELPHIA EAGLES would break their fifty-five-year drought and win the 2016 Super Bowl. Of course they did not, although if I could have seen the future and bet the farm that between 2017 and 2020 they would not only break that streak but become the first team in NFL history to win four Super Bowls in a row, well, I would be flying to the anniversary in my own private **Elon Musk*** electric jet that just went on sale for the bargain price of $2.5 million.

So, why the reluctance and cynicism? For those of you too young to remember, there was nothing optimistic about the future of healthcare delivery in 2016. In fact, no one was happy. We had spent years breaking the national bank by providing increasingly expensive high-tech care to those who were sick and could afford it. The model seems absolutely primitive by today's standards, where technology has advanced to the point that providers and patients work as a team to promote health in the workplace and at home. And while both care and caring have advanced beyond the wildest dreams of my 2016 self (we didn't even have implantable health chips back then), the real "failure" of the system was not in the lack of high-powered technology for diagnosis and treatment, but rather in the inability of the "humans" to work across specialties and disciplines, to hone their creativity and observation skills to partner with patients in advancing their health and to change course objectively, based on real-time data.

In fact, our failings started at the very beginning in how we chose and educated young physicians and nurses. Believe it or not, it's been less than ten years in which the MCATs (a multiple-choice test proving that an applicant can memorize organic chemistry formulas) was scrapped in favor of the now-national "empathy and self-awareness scale" that every aspiring physician or nurse recognizes as the most important "hurdle" they must overcome to be considered for medical school or nursing school admission. And it certainly came just in the nick of time, as I sit next to my robotic companion born from the Watson project. Simply put, I am no match for him/her/it when it comes to standard cognitive and memorization skills. But I can beat him/her/it hands down when it comes to comforting a patient or "reading between the lines" based on nuanced communication with a human patient.

---

* Elon Musk: a South African–born engineer, inventor, and investor. He conceptualized Mars Oasis (to build a greenhouse on Mars), Tesla Motors, and Solar City (to help combat global warming).

In fact, the only reason we "humans" are still needed as physicians is because we recognized in the nick of the time "what we bring to the table." We were never going to win the memorization or analytic war with our robotic computer counterparts. But, amazingly, that is how we chose physicians until a few short years ago. In other words, my ability to memorize complicated organic chemistry formulas meant that I had a leg up on remembering the nineteen reasons someone had a headache over the poor *schlub* who did not get into medical school because he/she could only remember fifteen. The fallacy in that old argument was just how easily a non–flesh-and-bones computer could replace that form of "us" by rattling off the differential diagnosis for any set of symptoms and then citing the references supporting the diagnosis, as well as a complete analysis of current treatment options—all in the time it takes me to put down my coffee and contemplate an answer.

There was a great set of movies about time travel almost forty years ago, largely forgotten, called *Back to the Future*, where one or two "aha moments" changed the course of history and set up alternate futures. And while many think the summit of healthcare leaders in 2016 changed the course of healthcare history, I believe it was simply math and uncommon sense.

The math was simple back in 2016 and pretty depressing. We wanted people to be healthy, but we counted on them being sick and using up lots of hospital beds. The real money flowed when people became sick—both profits and costs alike. I remember when I first took the job as an academic medical center president and chief executive officer (CEO). The very strong advice I got is that the two leadership jobs you didn't want to take in 2013 were in *academics* and *healthcare* because for both, the models that have existed for years are stale and impossibly unsustainable in the short term and fraught with pain in the longer term.

How stale and unsustainable was it? Back in 2016, a model entitled "fee for service" still reigned supreme—except there was no expectation of or guarantees of service or outcomes. In fact, it really should have been titled "fee for doing the things the healthcare provider decides you need and the more I do the more I get paid." And we were quite comfortable with that. Back in 2016, value was a futuristic concept and insurers, providers, and others spoke of moving "from volume to value." To be fair, some of the absurdities of the twentieth century were already being handled before the great summit of 2016. In that century, if I was a surgeon with a robust wound infection rate (perhaps because I did not wash my hands well enough), I earned more, in many cases, than a surgeon who followed careful guidelines. Because, believe it or not, there was a fee for the service of bringing you back to operate on the wound that was infected (in some cases, because of my improper technique).

That reward for failure was already being replaced with "pay for performance" and readmission penalties that at least did not *reward* poor technique and outcomes. In fact, the old math of the last century in healthcare has either been to promote and reward *overutilization* (volume) or some brief forays with promoting *underutilization* (managed care of the 1990s). One of the precepts that we take for granted now that was a direct outgrowth of the vapor-induced summit (more on the vapor part in a moment) of 2016 is that *optimal utilization*, which results in healthier populations, will be recognized and rewarded. As with so many logical ideas of 2026 (such as ending the *Rocky* franchise when **Sylvester Stallone** reached 75) that replaced bad ideas back in 2016 (not ending the **Kardashians'** TV reign soon enough), the concept of rewarding optimal utilization now seems as natural as stem cell hair replacement.

The old math plaguing healthcare is much older than the twentieth century and had its roots in the most fundamental precepts first described by **Euclid** in A.D. 300, when he described the unassailable facts regarding what later came to be known as Euclidian geometry. The fact Euclid recognized and articulated for the first time is that, as you think about a triangle, changing one angle—by definition—forces an inverse change in one of the other angles.

Fast-forward to 1970, when **William Kissick*** from the WHARTON SCHOOL OF BUSINESS at UNIVERSITY OF PENNSYLVANIA spoke of

---

*Iron Triangle: concept of healthcare first introduced in William Kissick's book *Medicine's Dilemmas: Infinite Needs Versus Finite Resources* in 1994. Kissick was also one of my professors at the WHARTON SCHOOL.

an "iron triangle of healthcare" around cost, access, and quality. As any ninth-grader versed in Euclidian geometry can tell you, if you increase an angle in said triangle, you need to decrease another. That translated to healthcare in this way. If you want to increase access, you need to increase cost or decrease quality. If you want to increase quality, you face either increased costs or decreased access . . . and so on.

The iron triangle is the Gordian knot of healthcare. It remains solid unless you take a sword to the geometry or, as **Einstein** said, "We can't solve problems by using the same kind of thinking we used when we created them." We needed to start thinking in terms of *fundamentally* transforming the *system* and changing the geometry, the way we think.

This challenge remained largely academic and festered under the surface until what is now known as the universal access bill of 2010 became law. At the time, it was called the Affordable Care Act. It wasn't affordable as it turns out and didn't do much to transform how care was delivered, but it did mandate near-universal access. The name was academic to its opponents (they called it Obamacare), many of whom wanted to go back to the "wondrous" days of the world's best healthcare system.

In fact, back in 2016, "we have the world's best healthcare system," easily rolled off the tongue of those whose interests were fortified by believing that statement. Conversely, "our public health parameters rank us among several third world countries while we pay for the world's most expensive system," countered those who wanted an extreme makeover. Undeniably, the national organization of America's healthcare system was marked by pessimism among graduating physicians, fear among hospital administrators who were not prepared to be judged based on a new value system, frustration by nurses and public health professionals, confusion by the public, and an almost slapstick melee between our legislators and executive branch, each arguing they knew what was best for the citizenry and finding real-life healthcare professionals (or at least actors wearing white coats) to support their positions.

Everyone, deep in their hearts, knew it even back then: The bubble needed to be burst and rebuilt into a much stronger and more sustainable structure. It just never happened. To create a new model for something as complicated and full of passion (and egos) as the American healthcare system would require *all* stakeholders to get together in a manner that had never been done before. But it never happened. Until January 2016.

Yes, I would love to say it was vision, amazing leadership, or an unprecedented level of collaboration between politicians and healthcare professionals. But that would be a lie . . . and revisionist history. And ever since the demise of Fox News and MSNBC, when people decided to stop being angry all the time and actually listen to other's opinions, facts have taken on a whole new level of importance in public discourse. So, the summit was born out of desperation, pure and simple.

President Obama realized that he had nothing to lose by calling together one last shot to preserve his legacy as the "healthcare president." I think what probably sent him over the edge (or at least got him to listen to the holographic **Harry Truman**) was the national presidential debates. At a time when healthcare was desperately in need of transformation and disruption, the cries of "Repeal Obamacare" and "Republicans Hate Women's Health" were about as creative as we got. So he rolled the dice. With the national debate regarding Obamacare roiling nearly six years after its passage and on the eve of a contentious national election, representatives of all major healthcare stakeholder groups were invited to a national conference on healthcare, appropriately called the "Last Big Shot at True Healthcare Reform at Big Sky" Summit, held in Montana.

Invited conference attendees/stakeholders in America's healthcare system included government representatives (state and federal), physicians (specialists and primary care), nurse and non-physician caregivers, public and population health professionals, hospital CEOs, insurance and payor leaders, employers (big and small), patients (acute, chronic, end of life), medical school and other healthcare school leaders (dean, faculty, student), pharmaceutical executives, medical device and information technology representatives, and attorneys (plaintiffs and defense). Fifty of the best and brightest (many of whom had many financial and other reasons to not fundamentally change the math that existed) were sent personal invitations by the president.

Why did everyone go along and decide to spend a weekend in Montana? Two individuals who chose *not* to attend the summit needed significant psychologic/psychiatric counseling to reconcile missing the most significant event of the twenty-first century (services that are much more easily obtained after the omnibus mental health tele-health act of 2018).

I think the real reason that almost everyone invited attended was that we were all tired of the almost universal pessimism about the future of healthcare. As one of my colleagues paraphrased **Woody Allen**, "We are at a crossroads—one road leads to total destruction, the other utter despair—let's hope we choose the right one." Not unlike all previous attempts to create a new model, this "last big shot summit" (which one of my more cynical colleagues called the "last *long* shot summit") initially went through the motions of tinkering around the edges talking about pay for performance models, bundled payments and accountable care organizations—all of which further exacerbated the depressing feeling that we were saving a system that needed to be scrapped and fanned the flickering hope that we might actually do something good.

CHAPTER 3

iPods, Interplanetary Travel, and What I Can Do to Transform Healthcare

A nd then it happened. As I think about it now, it reminds me of one of the crazy theories related to the genius and foresight of **Steve Jobs**. The theory goes something like this:

Steve was visited by interplanetary aliens in 1999, who gave him the idea for the iPod, iPhone, iPad, Apple watch, Apple Auto. And now Apple foods. (Yes, you now can get an APPLE apple—a genetically modified *Macintosh*, of course.) While I'm not sure why an alien race would have an interest in turning a failing computer company into the largest market cap corporation in the world dedicated to the digital age, the fact is that he/they did it (at least until INTERNATIONAL GENOMICS became the first $3 trillion market cap corporation in 2019). Jobs did it by assuming that the world *could* be fundamentally different in ten years and that APPLE could effect that change.

And so, the summit represented a "Jobsian" disruption in healthcare that, one could argue, has led us the 2026 healthcare that exists today; care that is affordable, universal, and easy to access with standardized quality and happy providers who embrace change and new technologies. Imagine if I had said that sentence ten years ago, prior to what is now called the optimistic healthcare revolution of 2016. "Hi, I envision healthcare that is affordable, universal, and easy to access with standardized quality and happy providers who embrace change and new technologies." An immediate drug test and psychiatric evaluation would have been the response of my colleagues back in 2016.

Whether it was a final act of our nation's 44th president, fatigue from all the pessimism, or just enough hope and optimism, the events of January 2016 have never been chronicled by someone who actually was there. This book serves as a memoir of what happened that fateful day when the parties involved in healthcare stopped talking about *reform* and what *others* should do—and started talking about *transformation* and the positive disruption that *"I"* can effect in creating an optimistic future in healthcare in America.

Who are we, your authors? We are the only participants who chose not to sign the confidentiality agreement after IT, THE BIG EVENT, happened—the confidentiality agreement that mandated you never talk about that day or what actually happened at the summit, other than the amazing outcome that came from the collaboration of the stakeholders, in exchange for a fair amount of dollars (again for you too young to remember, that was the nation's currency until the global bitcoin revolution of 2020 brought about by the fall of the Chinese economy).

One of us (**Steve Klasko**) is an obstetrician with an MBA from the WHARTON SCHOOL who had spent his pre-summit years doing research on physicians and what made them different than other people in how we handle change. Having watched so many of these meetings dissolve into acrimony, I was as skeptical about the outcome as anyone. But at the time, a week in Big Sky was a nice respite from the Euclidian geometry math that I was facing as a president of an academic medical center. And truth be told, I was not a first choice. The person who was supposed to represent academic medical centers decided it was a better use of time to keep a bicycle trip through Bordeaux, France, as opposed to participating in what would clearly be "another waste of time in healthcare policy."

One of us (**Greg Shea**) is a teacher and professor of organizational change who taught extensively at the ARESTY INSTITUTE OF EXECUTIVE EDUCATION and spent decades consulting, writing, and teaching about leadership and change. He was a "first choice" participant (well, his family wanted to believe so anyway) because of his predominant work in industries undergoing significant stress and change and assisting those stakeholders to think and act with the "system" in mind.

One is a journalist/writer (**Michael Hoad**) because someone needed to turn the proceedings into a readable document. **Anderson Cooper**, **Malcolm Gladwell**, even **Dr. Oz** all declined for unknown reasons (but probably because their careers would not be helped by being part of a very visible healthcare "failure"), so this person was chosen based on his work with the AAMC and a few academic medical centers in Florida and Pennsylvania that had the audacity to be optimistic about their future.

And finally, we were enormously helped by **Neil Gomes**, the youngest member of the summit. He had proven his "no limits" approach to utilizing technology to improve health and education through simulation, SECOND LIFE, and other modalities that, at the time, were groundbreaking.

So, that's us. The Beatles we were not. (For you post-millennials, the **Beatles** were a group of pre punk-rap musicians that have largely been forgotten since 2017). We aren't the **Rolling Stones** (who are still doing tours on the senior circuit), and we had not even heard of the **Four Zircons** who took **Daft Punk**'s banner forward and became the first truly robotic rock band to lead the digital charts. We simply believed enough to join what became the most *important* and the most *unusual* event of the first quarter of the twenty-first century.

Important: Because the twelve practical transformations outlined in these memoirs served as a basis for creating a new model in providing a healthier America—medically and economically. To quote **President Jenna Bush** (with thanks to **Buckminster Fuller**) during her inauguration speech in January 2021, "You never transform things by changing the existing reality; to transform healthcare in this country, we made a new reality that made the old way obsolete." That new reality updated and invigorated a very old aspiration articulated over a hundred years earlier by one of the founders of modern medicine, **William Osler**, "It is much more important to know what sort of a patient has a disease than what sort of a disease a patient has." That new/old reality paved the way for a collaborative healthcare environment where doctors work closely with nurses, clinical pharmacists, genomicists, healthcare coaches, and some of the newer providers trained through institutes of emerging health professions throughout the country—ranging from software engineers to sports and finance analytic experts to end-of-life counselors. And patients!

Unusual: Because of how THE EVENT happened. *It* happened quickly, like ripping off a Band-Aid. (Oh, I'm sorry. For those younger readers, a Band-Aid was an actual compression bandage invented by a woman who burned herself almost a hundred years before we counted on stem cell regeneration gels for healing.) Just as with other incremental changes in healthcare in the early twenty-first century, Band-Aids had "progressed" to having interesting images such as Superman (still making movies), Barbie (extinct), and **Duck Dynasty** (more on them later).

CHAPTER 4

AIR BNB* *or Am I Ready to Believe (Not Blame)*

And so we were summoned to a summit in Big Sky, Montana—by whom? The conference started typically enough (although, as we now know, very unusual occurrences birthed it). As usual, each stakeholder group expressed frustration with the failures of healthcare in America, the obstacles they face, and the obstructive, self-serving behavior consistent with an "it's everyone's fault but mine" mentality. The constipated and acrimonious nature of that discussion made me envy the CEO I replaced who decided not to attend and was probably just now parking her bicycle and sipping wine at CHÂTEAU MARGAUX.

Was it divine intervention?

Maybe.

Was it the same aliens that helped **Steve Jobs** develop a square box that would play 200 mp3s? (Again, a technology used before our current direct-to-brain digital form of post-media music expression.)

Possibly.

It was at least unusual and transformative. No one knows exactly what caused the blackout, but it had power behind it. What followed has euphemistically been called a UFO (unusually frank and open) discussion by some of the participants and as an act of God by religious leaders and at least one of the Republican legislators, but for us, we called it

---

*AIR BNB is a technology-enabled do-it-yourself movement for listing or renting lodging. But here, we're telling the story of a blackout that started a no blame conversation about healthcare. The consensus of this EVENT demanded a no blame model to build trust: "BNB Believe Not Blame."

what it was. The Great BNB, from "Believe Not Blame" because, some-how after the blackout and the strange vapor emanating into the room that caused all of us to lose consciousness for a second or two, a few very strange things happened.

First, there was a palpable energy surge among the participants, not unlike a collective jolt of a triple-venti latte.

But more importantly, the participants—those very same stake-holders who had, a few minutes before the UFO, alien, or divine inter-vention, blamed "everyone other than me" in a manner similar to the distributive arguments that framed the destructive healthcare debate around the Affordable Care Act—took a very different approach. From "it's the other person's fault" to "I am looking in the mirror and this is what I can do to transform healthcare," it was not unlike an old-time revival of spiritual awakening or a particularly emotional AA meeting.*

At the moment the parties involved in healthcare stopped talking about the difficulty and complexity of reform and what others should (but would never) do and started talking about transformation and the positive disruption *they* could effect in molding an optimistic future in healthcare in America, the ideas started flowing like water from a fire hose.

Forty-eight hours later, twelve practical transformations were de-veloped that served as a basis for creating a new model for a healthier America. That changed the entire healthcare presidential debate and became the platform (with a few minor differences) for *Both* the Demo-cratic and Republican parties.

For readers of my generation, here's a test: "Do you remember when **Donald Trump** was a leading contender for the Republican nomination for president?" So, the chance that a national consensus on anything about healthcare would have seemed as likely ten years ago as three gen-dered aliens abducting a medical student in order to help her understand

---

*Studies show that consensus is broken by a lack of trust, especially when there is unequal power among the participants in a dialogue: Stanley Deetz and Jennifer Simpson (2003) "Critical Organizational Dialogue," in Dialogue: Theorizing Differ-ence, edited by Anderson, Baxter, Cissna.

the business of medicine (a subject of a former book written by us). I fully acknowledge, however, that for the students and younger readers of these memoirs, the preceding statement is an absolute "so what." "Healthcare and universal access and population health is not a debatable topic, and the parties find other things to fight about. Who is going to argue about improving the access, quality, and cost of keeping the population healthier?" they might say and ask. For those of us who lived the dark days of **Sean Hannity** vs. **Rachel Maddow,*** it is every bit as fundamental a transformation as moving from treating cancer based on the organ of origin in the pre-genomic days or actually having to go to an airport to board a plane in the pre–self-guided personal aircraft days.

History matters, and the purpose of the following pages is to chronicle the forty-eight-hour discussion and, most importantly, the precepts that have come to be known as the "Dozen Disruptors for the Demise of the Old Healthcare."

Transtemporal angel induced, alien induced, drug induced, or divine: Whatever you call the twelve precepts, it doesn't matter. Thanks to them, we now take for granted as part of our everyday "healthier" lives the fact that healthcare in America is logical, easy to access, consumer-driven, and, most importantly, dynamically changing based on technology, logic, creativity, science, *and* human interaction.

What are the precepts? On what do they rest? How did they arise? Read on.

---

*Hannity and Maddow: Sean Hannity (Fox) and Rachel Maddow (MSNBC) who epitomize the cable news format of "Let me watch something that will just get me angrier and more strident about an issue I am already pretty angry and strident about."

CHAPTER 5

Overcoming Inertia, Icebergs, and Iron Triangles

A No-Blame VAPOR Strikes THE EVENT*

The summit, THE EVENT, began with a flash. We didn't know if it was a blackout, a vapor, or even a loss of consciousness. It caused confusion, but no panic and a short period of discussion about electricity grids, terrorism, and Chinese hackers passing as residents of Des Moines. Fortunately, the computers were still working and the coffee was even still hot, so we all got back to work. The changes started subtly, and it took a while for us to understand that something special was happening in this lodge in the middle of Montana.

As luck (or fate) would have it, the topic immediately preceding the blackout was about the high cost of defensive medicine and the impact of malpractice on healthcare and healthcare costs. Right before the blackout, the panel consisting of a plaintiff lawyer, a malpractice defense lawyer, one Republican and one Democratic senator, and a neurosurgeon were talking *at* each other about the "evils of the current system that victimize the providers" (neurosurgeon) or the "fact that someone has to stand up for the victims of medical errors and, by the way, the fact

---

*VAPOR: A fog that drifted through the conference (the EVENT) causing all of us to adopt a blame-free dialogue. Without the VAPOR, we would have descended into accusation. But we never figured out where it came from, or who engineered its presence.

*The EVENT: An invited conference at Big Sky, where the participants were affected by a VAPOR that made possible the kind of exchange envisioned by Presidents Barack Obama and Harry Truman.

that I have two citation jets is beside the point and a cheap shot" (personal injury attorney to the AMA rep).

Then the vapor hit as we heard background music, **Warren Zevon's** "Lawyers, Guns, and Money" leading into **Tom Waits'** "Step Right Up." Who was in charge of the music?

It was then that the not-so-subtle changes began. Awaiting more fireworks related to "it's about the greedy lawyers" or "its about the incompetent doctors," the defense attorney got up and made a statement that I would later realize began the healthcare revolution/evolution of 2016. "I believe we can come to an agreement on principles, not positions. We all learned about collaborative negotiations in college and graduate school,"* he stated.

I was going to interrupt and say that, as a physician trained in the twentieth century, we did not learn any of that because we could not afford to take any precious time away from learning microbiology, biochemistry, etc., to dabble in mundane exercises like learning how to negotiate and communicate.

> I am sure my professors knew what was best for me when they decided that it was more important for me to understand the citric acid cycle, in which three equivalents of nicotinamide adenine dinucleotide (NAD^+) into three equivalents of reduced NAD^+ (NADH), one equivalent of flavin adeninine dinucleotide (FAD) into one equivalent of $FADH_2$, and one equivalent each of guanosine diphosphate (GDP) and inorganic phosphate (P_i) into one equivalent of guanosine triphosphate (GTP). Or, I kid you not, I had to memorize this formula:

$$CH_3C(=O)C(=O)O- + HSCoA + NAD+ \rightarrow$$
$$CH_3C(=O)SCoA \text{ (acetyl-CoA)} + NADH + CO_2$$

Anyhow, the defense attorney continued. "What if we get back to basics: positions, issues, and interests. We have been stuck during this conference (and I would say during the last fifty years) on *positions*—greedy lawyers, incompetent doctors. While that may be true in a small

---

* Throughout this book, the quotations are real.

minority of the cases, that is not where the solution is. The solution is looking at *issues* and *interests* of the parties involved and of all of the relevant stakeholders."

"Right. And what if we actually thought about what we want this thing called the American healthcare system to do? What do we want from it?"

So, as the old adage goes, I realized I was "not in Kansas anymore."

In fact, while I was in the same physical conference room as before, I was not even in the same virtual universe that I remembered before the blackout because everything had changed.

The physician got up to the whiteboard and asked the personal injury attorney to join him. "Let's create a bargaining iceberg looking at solutions around principles regarding malpractice and bad medical events. For those of you not acquainted with negotiation theory, we are right here." He pointed to the very tip of the iceberg and labeled it *positions*. I am going to stand here with my colleague who has devoted his career to standing up for victims of what he perceives to be malpractice."

Now I knew I wasn't in Kansas any more and something real was changing.

He continued, "and together we are going to see if there are common issues and interests that we can agree upon on behalf of the people we represent."

They both started writing. On the block labeled "issues," the plaintiff attorney confidently and hurriedly wrote, "allowing patients who have been harmed access to the malpractice legal system without undue hurdles." The counselor for the defense, after contemplating a few different answers, wrote in a slightly less emphatic manner, "reducing poor outcomes through technology and training."

Then the fun began, a different kind of fun than before the blackout. That kind of fun was like watching old reality TV shows (remember the allusion to **Duck Dynasty**) where it was fun watching people yell and scream at each other. This kind of fun was very different, more like listening to a perfect three-tenor harmony. All five panelists and a few people from the audience started writing on the board.

Finally, the AMA representative looked and said, "While those issues are interesting and true, they represent parallel thinking and do not help us necessarily get to an answer. But reading some of the comments, at least the ones I can read" (a clear allusion to the docs' bold but almost illegible handwriting), "I believe we may have some common interests that could lead to some principles for a solution." He then started walking around the board, stroking his chin. If he had a pipe, I would have envisioned him as a modern day **Sherlock Holmes** contemplating an especially difficult case. "Here's how I would summarize the interests we share." The cynical side of me wondered if "interests we share" had ever been used in the same sentence between doctors and lawyers talking about malpractice. But I continued to virtually pinch myself and listen.

"Here is what I believe we've all agreed upon as shared interests," he continued looking directly at me (or maybe I was feeling guilty about my negative thoughts at this time of awakening).

"First, we need to promote the reduction of medical errors. We need to truly reward and herald best practices, such as zero percent wound infection rates, and proselytize the processes that allowed those zero defects to happen. Then we need to educate and remediate physicians who have room to improve. We need to look at the human component to quality breakdowns."

It actually all made sense. At first I was mesmerized by the simple elegance of the argument. My next emotion was one of frustration based on recognizing what could have happened if we had been willing to have these discussions long ago. By the time I was ruminating, lamenting, and contemplating, the rest of the board had been filled with this logic:

Human Component to Quality Breakdowns

Human error—inadvertently doing other than what should have been done: slip, lapse, mistake

At-risk behavior—behavior that increases risk where risk is not recognized or is mistakenly believed to be justified

Reckless behavior—choice to consciously disregard a substantial and unjustifiable risk

One of the chief medical officers from the audience jumped on the stage and said, "You know, I've had it all wrong. If I look at it this way, I have to fundamentally change my response. In some respects, a human error from one of the docs on my medical staff is *my* fault because we should create system designs that minimize those chances. Those physicians should be consoled, not punished, and change should be mediated through processes, procedures, training, design, and environment."

He continued, "I would call your at-risk behavior cohort more like unintentional risk-taking. Those physicians and providers need to be coached. I should be responsible for doing that through removing incentives for at-risk behaviors, creating incentives for healthy behaviors, and increasing situational awareness for the entire staff. This way, I can reserve *punishment* for that reckless group, the intentional risk takers, through remedial and disciplinary action. I believe we can all agree on the need to remove and/or retrain reckless providers."

The base of the bargaining iceberg was filled in quickly. "We have to allow patients to get appropriate relief of harm related to medical errors. I think we all agree we need a national debate on appropriate relief and appropriate lawyer's fees after expenses."

OK, I thought, here is where the harmony ends. But I was wrong. The lawyers and doctors nodded in unison like one of those old bobble head dolls that used to adorn people's automobiles.

"We need to remove the disparities between counties and states as to guidelines and relief. And we need to educate patients both about the need to ask proper questions and the effect of our current malpractice system on their care."

And there it was. The first example that something different really was happening. That the blackout was not an electrical grid, alien invasion, or Chinese hacking problem. It was the beginning of the rational revolution in healthcare, the BNB—Believe Not Blame.

✦ ✦ ✦

The following two hours went by like a blur with almost everyone in the audience looking at what *they* could do to fundamentally alter a broken malpractice-defensive medicine vicious cycle. One of the ideas was so easy and so logical (and so obvious today) that there was an almost audible collective sigh when it was proposed.

It actually came from the Chief Information Officer (CIO) of a top twenty academic medical center whose first career had been to develop supply chain systems for HOME DEPOT. "Think about this: When I was in industry, almost any interaction we have with a customer is recorded, ostensibly for customer service purposes, but also to have a legal and documented record. But in healthcare, informed consent is often given in a closed room, and the patient signs a standardized preprinted form with the procedure and potential complications scribbled in. There is no record of what was actually said in the room. Should the patient have a complication, second thoughts, or any other reason to be angry, she can sue the physicians, and the only record of the informed consent is either her or the doctor's perception of what happened in that room, usually with the degradation of memory brought on by the few years it took to get to trial."

He stopped for a minute and went over to the defense attorney on the stage. "What did you have for breakfast on August 12, 2012?"

"I assume that's a rhetorical question . . . unless there is something special about that date. If you want I can guess what I usually have," was the very logical reply.

"Aha, that's exactly right," said the CIO. "Which is exactly what happens on the witness stand. The attorney for the plaintiff will make the case that the informed consent was inadequate, which will be bolstered by the plaintiff during her testimony. She will make it sound like the doctor spent twenty *seconds* with her and she had no understanding of what was being done, what the alternatives were, or what potential complications might ensue. If she had known all that, she will aver, then she never would have consented to the procedure. Fast-forward to the doctor's testimony, and his recollection is that he spent twenty *minutes* painstakingly going through the procedure, its alternatives, and potential complications. Is either of them lying? Not really. Any more than you would be if you were forced to remember what you ate for breakfast on any given date several years ago. But because we all seem to be looking in the mirror now, I am embarrassed that I didn't formulate the software and technology solution to *this* problem before."

What the "*this*" was became a theme in the post-BNB discussions that took place. Why couldn't we use at least the technology that is used at HOME DEPOT or other retailers for customer service and legal reasons when a customer calls about returning an electric drill, to record the patient–physician interaction when a doctor is proposing opening up a patient's abdomen? Why can't we attach it to the record and not have to guess in a courtroom what was said in that closed room several years later? Why has healthcare somehow escaped the consumer logic that every other retail and consumer organization has evolved to?

Once again, the panel perked up and, almost in unison, ideas started to flow from the attorneys, physicians, and information technology folks. The standard that is used today in 2026 is a direct outgrowth of that vibrant and logical discussion.

Today, in 2026, a physician would not dream of doing an informed consent without the benefit of the encounter being recorded. In fact, almost immediately after the Montana EVENT was over in 2016, the president created a council of attorneys (defense and plaintiff) and physicians to come up with the ideal informed consent for the top fifty procedures performed in the United States. These were printed and recorded in seven languages and sent to every physician and physician's office in the country.

Today, a patient who will need a procedure is counseled by a nurse or physician assistant regarding the procedure. The pre-authorized and pre-blessed informed consent is read to the patient after a quick reminder, "We will be recording this so we and you have documentation of this encounter." The informed consent is read, and the patient verbally agrees and signs the document. The physician then comes in and answers any questions that were not addressed, and the patient goes home. Sometime before the procedure, the patient needs to review a video, relook at the informed consent, and—on her APPLE tele-health monitor, or GOOGLE Glass, or old-school home computer—answer a few multiple-choice questions such as:

The three most common complications of my procedure are . . .

The alternatives to having this done are . . .

The last question would be:

> I understand the procedure, its complications, and the alternatives
> and I am ready to proceed . . . true or false.

Back in 2016, the CIO emphatically put the microphone down, and the thud was not unlike a thunderbolt to the audience—not because the idea was so brilliant, but because the concept was so logical, so easy.

"Why didn't we do this before?" a senator from Pennsylvania got up and almost seemed angry. "It seems that healthcare has somehow escaped the consumer revolution, the information technology revolution, and several other lesser revolutions. Why did it take this event, whatever it is that happened to us, for us to come up with these simple, logical, and agreed upon solutions?"

For the first time since the blackout, there seemed to be some anger in the room. "I think it's funny that a member of the same party that brought us Obamacare would be lecturing to us about logic and simplicity," was the comment from the chair of oncology of a community hospital in Georgia. In almost mid-sentence, he stopped talking and clutched his head. One of the apparent side effects of the BNB VAPOR was the sudden onset of a splitting headache if the "NB—not blame" was breached.

Time for a reception!

Changes 2016–2026

What's Changed the Most in Malpractice Prevention and Quality Control in 2026?

1. Informed consent is no longer a closed-door, individual exercise, but rather a standardized, recorded, and understandable counseling format.

2. Quality is assumed and transparent. All negative outcomes are included on a decision support database, which helps to guide future practice.

3. Malpractice cases are triaged by an impartial panel of physicians and attorneys. Cases deemed to be poor outcomes are arbitrated; ones felt to have negligence components are tried.

What Happened in 2016 That Led to the Transformation?

1. Millennials expected to have the same ability to compare doctors and hospitals as they do to compare restaurants and hotels.

2. The "zero defect expectation" became one of the outgrowths of the conference. Physicians were no longer "rewarded" just for having fewer mistakes or hospital-acquired infections than the previous year.

3. Non-profit CEOs were mandated to have their incentives match the organization's vision and include cost, access, and quality.

CHAPTER 6

Getting *From* Here *To* There

From Fear and Opacity
to Optimism and Transparency

There is no better way to defuse tension than to turn emotion into an academic exercise. And that is exactly what **Greg** was able to accomplish in turning around this emotional response to one that allowed the process to continue.

He started with a simple statement: "Rather than be upset that the medical system you knew was disturbed, you should be amazed that it took this long. Simply put, you allowed an inefficient, expensive, inconsistent system to exist for way too long, and it was bound to end eventually. But you now have a great opportunity to not only change how you deliver healthcare but how you view the *systems* that drive health. I have spent my career working with other industries to design systems that are consistent and not left to the vagaries of the individual. It just makes sense that something as important as the health of an individual and population should use the same system approach that has reduced errors in supply chain and manufacturing."

The patient advocate piled on: "I recently had an elective procedure at my local hospital, and despite my PhD, I was not one of the lucky few that could make any sense out of the bill I was sent or what I was actually purchasing. If you don't want to tackle that problem, try sorting out funds flow for support of medical education. Or attempt to establish the cost of producing a drug or medical device or any rational basis for its price once it's approved. Perhaps hardest of all, we spent a fair amount of time earlier talking about optimal utilization and rewarding quality.

I can understand the parameters for a quality grade in most other areas of the economy, but to this point, measuring what quality of care really means to a patient has eluded the healthcare industry, and we have been left with some very imperfect grading systems."

The consultant attempted a summary, "What we can all agree on, past history and blame aside, is that we have failed to determine reproducible and consistent quality parameters, to work with the government and private sector to rationalize the sources and uses of funds for medical education, to demand transparency in drug pricing, or to just plain have enough respect for patients to rectify the absurd way that people are billed for what happens in a hospital or doctor's office."

I regrouped just in time to see the patient lean forward, "In the spirit of post-blackout BNB, and as someone who can speak as a patient and a consultant for the industry, there is blame all around. We patients have not demanded anywhere near the level of transparency we demand in the rest of our lives. To make matters worse, healthcare providers have been, well, lazy, or at least have not felt a burning platform."

"That's not fair," the primary care physician interrupted. "We absolutely are passionate about caring for every patient we see."

"That is true," the entrepreneur continued, "and the genius of American medicine has been the focus on the individual. But, by definition, that makes you a poor allocator of resources."

The patient advocate chimed in. "In our new spirit of looking in the mirror, the same is true of patients. Everyone would like managed care that reduces costs for everyone other than themselves and their family. For them and their family, they want everything, cost be damned, as long as someone else is paying for it. No matter who you blame, whether it is someone else or ourselves, the components of the healthcare system don't allow for access, quality, and cost to be maximized. It is like a beautiful car but the parts don't fit into the design!" exclaimed the congressman who had, heretofore, been pretty silent (and was indeed a car dealer).

CHAPTER 7

Healthcare Systems
and Homo Sapiens

I felt the heat rising in the room and the newfound spirit of blamelessness under siege. A professor then offered a useful, if slightly long-winded, perspective. Recognizing that this would require even more introspection, he offered a thought: "I don't want to speak too long, so I will give you some homework."

"Some things even supernatural events can't change!" the congressman continued.

"That's because you are thinking of the components and not the system," the professor continued, speaking to all of us.

The health policy expert seemed to have an epiphany. "If I may, healthcare qualifies not just as a system, but as a particularly complicated system. It mixes market forces with government subsidies and a multitude of regulations and licensing procedures covering institutions, as well as those they employ or with whom they contract."

The cool thing about post-vapor discussions was that, almost like synchronized swimming, participants actually listened to others and then added their thoughts.

The neurosurgeon put it in clinical terms: "The work of caring for people is complex enough because Homo sapiens amount to a complex system of complex systems themselves, biologically and emotionally. Those complicated systems mean that a lot can go wrong, even though our bodies do a remarkable job of keeping us functioning. We adapt and compensate in a most impressive fashion, but our mind and bodies (I'll leave our souls out of it for now) do have lots of so-called moving parts that can and do get damaged, break, or simply wear out. Caring for humans grows ever more complicated as our capabilities to repair and replace just about anything improve dramatically—thanks to scientific, technological, and clinical advances—as well as to the wealth in our society and its willingness and ability to pay for healthcare. In America, we then make caring for people still more complicated (and frustrating) through byzantine processes and de facto and de jure informational firewalls."

"Got it, I think! Then all of this combines to enable and indeed to reward finger-pointing and deflection—hence, our entire pre-blackout history of American healthcare," was a thoughtful response from one of the health policy experts.

The health policy expert: "So, because (at least post-blackout and BNB) we are looking for solutions, not just definitions of problems, what would happen if we break this cycle? In other words, if we didn't collude, if we weren't partners in creating these inefficient systems? Just what will that new world look like, what would it involve, and how will it evolve? It would be too easy to just say we need to 'go APPLE' and 'think different.' So, to get from theory to practice, more precisely, we will need to think systemically and to help others to think that way as well.

"To notably improve healthcare in the United States, we should think about healthcare as a system, understand it as a system, and fix it as a system. Trying to mend one component, pushing here or pulling there, may provide a moment of emotional release or garner a few votes or prop up revenues, but changing a piece seldom changes a system. The altered piece eventually snaps back into its former dysfunctional place.

"In other words, **President Obama** had it right when he promised repeatedly that he would gather those stakeholders who represented the many and various pieces of the healthcare system (that would be all of you) and broadcast live the negotiations to reform it. You don't believe me, when you are back in the real world try this YouTube link (www.youtube.com/watch?v=akVkzm0YPAc)." YouTube, for those of you not interested in remembering a decade ago, was a relatively primitive attempt to disseminate video content prior to the development of implantable optical video chips, the internet of things and ALL-FLIX.

The policy expert concluded: "Finally, such an approach would have put the *system* on display and shown the finger-pointing for what it was and is: misdirection. Such an approach would have also encapsulated the system for the examination and education of all. So, actually President Obama had it right, and then he changed his mind. Until now!"

It is almost hard to fathom an audience of physicians and pharma and insurance executives being lectured to about their failings and turning Obamacare from a legislative achievement or a nightmare (courtesy of MSNBC and Fox) to a wake-up call for a healthcare system that, up until 2016, had been saddled with pessimism and lethargy.

"OK, I get it." An invited neurosurgeon provided the first comment in what had been an uncontested and uninterrupted combination of look to the future and rebuke of the past. "So, I want to be optimistic. Sounds like fun. So I'll drink the Kool-Aid, or probably more accurately inhale the vapor. But how do we convert inevitable change to optimism?"

A sly smile preceded the reply. "Hanging on to how you did things before is easy. Change requires energy. Energy can come from fear, to be sure. Threatened, we can rush to protect and to defend. Our anxiety climbs as our intelligence falls. Our explanations become simpler and our emotions more primitive. Our minds close (and our sphincters tighten). Our actions grow more punitive and simple minded even as they grow in intensity. 'Burning platforms' cause us to change by making us first jump around and then just jump, and fear becomes the fuel of choice. Once expended though, this fuel leaves behind exhaustion. The mother who picks the car off her infant does not simply pick up her child and her bundles and head off to her next adrenaline-soaked superhuman adventure.

"Optimism (usually not used in the same sentence as healthcare for the four decades up until 2016), especially when tied to a dream or hope for a better future, can provide a very different fuel that can be either used on its own or mixed with fear. **Martin Seligman**, for example, built on the work of **Aaron Beck** and demonstrated the power of optimism and the potential to develop it."*

---

* By the way, current 2026 readers, even though we have come a long way in fixing these problems over the past ten years, the vigilance needed to maintain a rational system will require continued surveillance by all the stakeholders reading this book.

Optimism and its cousin *hope* can also fuel change. The dynamics differ from fear because, unlike fear, optimism and hope take longer to learn and develop, especially in the more experienced, even jaded among us. Developing the "pull" of a dream differs from injecting the "push" born of fear of the present or uncertain future. Dreams pull people along, but often arise from humble and stumbling beginnings, requiring small, quick wins to avoid being stillborn.

Other sources of positive energy for change include a sense of meaning and a "winning attitude." It sounds trite, but research has long shown the connection between job satisfaction and the sense of contributing to something larger—one's group, the organization, or a grander purpose. "That's probably why academic physicians have always tolerated a lower salary and significantly more hassles than their private colleagues in exchange for being part of a greater 'faculty,'" said the dean, almost seeming as if he was trying to convince himself.

"True," you bring up the operative point. "Positive energy for change argues for clarity of role and of vision or, at least knowing what one is to do and why it matters. Overcoming threats, in and of itself, can provide that sense of satisfaction, but it's only a temporary fix. Helping to move toward a better world can also provide a sense of satisfaction and the related energy to keep going. That energy can last longer than can spikes of fear, but it depends on connection of self to a larger purpose and ongoing indications of progress that reinforce the optimism that the dream is in fact possible."

"It sounds like it's a pretty thin line between optimism and delusion. I know that a lot of people have made a lot of money writing books and giving lectures on the importance of a winning attitude. But, by itself, it seems worthless because it can make us numb to feedback and slow to learn," offered the nurse practitioner, giving an example of the $5 million in consultant fees that had been spent in her health system to "change the culture" with minimal results.

The professor ended with a thought that had everyone scratching their heads (and heading for the bar!): "The secret sauce, according to lots of research on goals and achievement, is the ability to develop demanding, consequential, but achievable goals. Telling the woefully underqualified that they can accomplish anything that they put their minds to sets them (and the leader) up for failure, no matter how many inspiring consultants you bring in. Wins produce a grounded and maintainable winning attitude. They feed optimism and support dreams."

So—and I know this was the long way around to getting here, but I am an academic physician, so part of my job is to take a long time to get to a simple conclusion—the simple conclusion for us is this. When we leave Montana and try to convince our "non-vaporized" colleagues of this optimistic future, we are in for a long and arduous trek. And long treks, of which systemic healthcare reform certainly qualifies, require you to walk toward a dream, not run from a fear. "Eating large items one bite at a time" is an apt metaphor for assigning roles and connecting them through challenging but achievable goals to a larger purpose. So, we will need to concentrate on producing visible wins, especially in the beginning, no matter how small. Tenacity can slip into stubbornness and then into outright pigheadedness. But visible wins utilizing a different mindset are the best antidote. Failure to think systems, in other words, helps to generate emotions that can feel good even as they inhibit change. Systems thinking and problem solving (or non–systems thinking and counterproductive blaming) comprise the platform on which this whole conference rests.

"When you get back to your rooms, there will be some homework on systems thinking well worth reading," the professor concluded.*

And so it went. Lecture over. Homework assigned. One day down. It was now midnight and what started like a wasted weekend was slowly beginning to feel like the beginning of a revolution—a bloodless revolution fueled by optimism, systems thinking, and concentrating on the patients, providers, and students of the future instead of pretending that we can justify or continue the past.

Overnight, no rest for the weary.

---

* For readers of the book following along, please see "Homework Assignments" at the end of the narrative.

CHAPTER 8

Let My Perceptions Go

Ten Commandments and a Dozen Disruptors

I woke up the next morning in a fog. It was one of those surreal mornings where it took me a full fifteen minutes of wakefulness to decide if all of yesterday was a dream or not. It wasn't. And I woke up singing an old **Beach Boys** song, "Wouldn't It Be Nice" (if you are too young to know that group, listen to it—you'll thank me).

The anticipation of what could possibly happen on the second day of the conference overcame any skepticism of whether or not this vapor-induced "what can I do to fundamentally transform healthcare" mentality would last or whether yesterday was equivalent to a one-hit wonder (remember the **Tom Tom Club**). Back at the summit, would we go back to our blaming mentality: "I'm OK, you're not."

The answer came quickly and before I had a chance to even smell the latte. Right at the entrance to the conference room, at a small table, was the medical director from an elite Ivy League institution, a patient advocate, and a small business CEO enjoying their omelets and having an animated conversation that would have been inconceivable several years ago, even a month ago—hell, even twenty-four hours ago.

It went something like this. The medical director started: "I feel bad. We as an industry have abandoned you during the consumer revolution. How come you can do really cool things in every area of your life: holiday shopping on your iPhone or Android, for example, or arrange travel through a variety of e-apps, but you still have to access the healthcare system like you did in the nineties?"

She looked at him and said in a reassuring tone that would have been impossible in the pre-BNB universe, "Look, we as patients and employers deserve some responsibility also. I can't tell you how many times I have been frustrated by the system but rather than complain or change providers, I let it go because I figured, that's healthcare, nothing I can do about it."

She started to get angry, and then in just a second began to smile. It was hard to tell whether the change in emotion was reflection or a product of the lingering effects of the vapor and blackout. "Let me give you two examples that actually happened to me and my family. One of them was several years ago, at your hospital as a matter of fact." The physician executive barely perceptibly raised his eyebrows. She continued, in almost a sad tone, "If healthcare were any other business, and what I am about to tell you were commonplace, you would be out of business."

"Is it too early for a Bloody Mary? I have a feeling I am going to need one," the medical officer did elicit a chuckle from that.

"No, I'm confident you will be able to handle the criticism. Thanks to our alien or divine vapor and intervention, I believe you will make fundamental changes after this weekend," she said emphatically.

"I went to your hospital for a women's health exam. I had a mammogram, and the technician was clearly uncomfortable with the results and went on to explain, with what she probably believed was a sympathetic tone, that I will probably need magnification views because something doesn't seem right. I innocently asked when she thought I would know the results. And in a straight voice, she said that it would take about a week, explaining to me that the radiologists like to batch read (I've come to realize that means that they don't want to bother reading the mammograms until there are enough to read). They would then read the mammogram and dictate a report and get it to my doctor's office. Then it was a roll of the dice as to when they would decide to call me (my words, not the technician's)."

"Now I know this is going to sound sarcastic, but what happened next was quite spontaneous and quite sincere. I saw about ten feet away what I assumed was the radiologist, so I said, 'there's a guy with a white coat over there drinking coffee who looks suspiciously like a radiologist. Is there any reason he couldn't take a look at this?' The technologist was both surprised and responsive. After a few minutes in conversation with the radiologist, he sauntered over, introduced himself, and spent the next two minutes looking at the digital image. He then moved his gaze to me and said, 'Your mammogram is perfectly normal. See you in a year.'"

"OK, good outcome then, so you should be happy, right?" the physician sitting next to her barely stopped eating his waffle to ask that insightful question.

"Well, yes as a matter of fact, I was at first, but then it hit me that it was only because I asked the question and because the radiologist agreed to walk the ten feet, that I went home reassured as opposed to being sleepless for several nights waiting for an archaic process to play out. I know there are some places that guarantee same day results . . . but dammit, it ought to be the standard, not the exception."

"I'll see your absurd story and raise you one," I had barely noticed the middle-aged man sitting next to me wearing a TAMPA BAY BUCS pin. "So, I run a small business in Florida and I was looking for the right place to go to get my mother tested for memory loss. My dad had Alzheimer's and passed away, and now my mom is worried that she might be in the early stages. I was hoping it was just stress on my mom from losing her husband, but I figured it was worth checking. Fortunately, we live close to the state-funded Alzheimer's and memory disorders center. So, I called. Believe it or not, for Florida's MEMORY DISORDER CENTER, the access message asks you to 'please listen to the following eleven options before you make your choice.' My first reaction was, how brilliant. They can screen out who really needs them. If you can actually figure out how to get an appointment, your memory must be OK. But then, just like you, I got angry and frustrated. I realized its just healthcare—a *Saturday Night Live* version of customer service!" He started to laugh at his own story. But he was right. It is cartoonish that we cannot get this customer service thing right.

Breakfast was over. Rather than a bell or a buzzer, music started playing, and instinctively, the invited guests began milling into the conference room.

That music again—what a playlist! Whoever was organizing the conference had an interesting sense of humor. Today's time to get started selections included "Skating Away on the Thin Ice of a New Day" by **Jethro Tull**, "Don't Stop Believing" by **Journey**, "Who's Gonna Take the Blame" by **Smokey Robinson and the Miracles**, "Everything Has Changed" by **Taylor Swift**, and "Time Has Come Today" by the **Chambers Brothers**. Putting musical taste aside, it did not go unnoticed that not-so-subtle signals were being sent that today was going to be different.

Perhaps the oddest "post-vapor" aspect of the conference is that every participant instinctively started filling up the seats from front to back. Now that might not seem so odd to anyone who doesn't go to many healthcare or academic conferences, but at least for doctors, it is an almost unwritten rule that the back fills up first. I always wondered as I was giving talks in large auditoriums why the first few rows were always empty. It never made any sense to me, it was like it was SEA WORLD and **Shamu** was going to be drenching anyone naïve enough to inhabit the front.

I was woken from my meaningless musing with a warning about a very different animal. "There is an elephant in the room." A tall, square-jawed woman who looked familiar was now up on the stage talking. "It seems to me that yesterday was the ultimate wake-up call, and now that we seem to be incapable of retreating to the comfort of blaming everyone else for our inefficiencies, customer non-centricity, and quality control in healthcare—the question becomes what do we do. Blaming *ourselves* is no better than where we were before where we blamed *everyone else* if it doesn't lead to a prescription for a new healthcare that is transformative, yet achievable and logical."

Almost universal nodding emerged from the front rows, which were filled and nearly silent.

The person next to her, a very scholarly looking bow-tied man I hadn't noticed until that moment, interrupted. "Baby steps," he said. "We need to consider the art of the possible. Inch by inch we can start to get this right."

The first speaker started to get angry, but then just smiled. (I guess the BNB vapor was still having its effect). "Look, I was the CEO of one of the world's largest airline companies, and we became a breakout success once we started to think about what it will take to satisfy the customers of the future because the present becomes the past pretty quickly and your success can fade just as quickly." I remembered her now from one of those annoying messages you hear as you are about to take off on a flight from the CEO of the airline you were about to take off on. But she was about to "take off" on an approach to transformation of healthcare that would have all of us "fastening our seat belts."

"I couldn't disagree with you more about baby steps and the art of the possible. The time for incremental steps is over. However this unlikely series of events that led us here happened, we have been given an opportunity to change the plan and do the *impossible*. I graduated from UNIVERSITY OF MICHIGAN and shared the stage with **Larry Page*** at the 2009 commencement, and he made a comment that was very GOOGLE-like but could not be more relevant for today. He said that he thought it is often easier to make progress on mega-ambitious dreams. Because no one else is crazy enough to do it, you have little competition. In fact, 'there are so few people this crazy that I feel like I know them all' by first name."

She stopped for a moment and became deadly serious. "I don't know what happened yesterday, but it certainly was a disruptive event. But, frankly if all we do is look in the mirror and blame ourselves for the lack of creativity in healthcare delivery, we will have accomplished nothing. This is like one of those science fiction movies where we get to start a new world knowing everything we need to know about the past but not being bound by it."

Dr. "Bow-tie" (he was actually the longest standing dean of a medical college in the country and seemed to come from central casting, Cambridge, academics, Ivy League) said, "OK, then let's get started. Perhaps we could quote someone equally as visionary for his time, but a bit more academic. I believe that **Buckminster Fuller** got it right when he said that 'you never change things by fighting the existing

---

*Larry Page: GOOGLE founder who also said, "If your access to healthcare involves your leaving work and driving somewhere and parking and waiting for a long time, that's not going to promote healthiness."

reality. To change something, build a new model that makes the existing model obsolete.' So you are right, the hell with baby steps, lets leap into the future. We almost need a ten commandments for the new healthcare that can serve as a blueprint for our new transformed world of healthcare."

A tall, thin, thirty-something man shot up and said, "Sounds great, but if I could be so bold, **Moses** got it right for his time. But for the twenty-first century, let's bag the stone tablets, because this will need to be a living, breathing blueprint. Besides, ten commandments sounds a little proscriptive and stuffy to me. I was never good with authority and never really reacted well to what I shalt and shalt not do. I think we go with a new concept: Let's create a dozen disruptors for the future of healthcare."

Readers, that's how it happened. Book one of the genesis of the new healthcare. What came to be known as the D-5, "Disruptive Dozen Dimensions of a Dramatically Different Healthcare for America"* started with that innocent comment. No burning bushes, stone tablets, and certainly no days of rest. We went right to work.

"Here is what I suggest. It turns out that randomly" (although nothing seemed to be random nowadays, almost everything felt like a grand design, but whose?), "there is a representative stakeholder of each aspect of the healthcare system sitting on the aisle of every row. Don't ask me how I know that. If you haven't suspended disbelief by now, you never will.

"Looking at the aisles, I see a government representative, a physician, a nurse practitioner, a population health professional, a patient advocate, a community advocate, a health system CEO, and insurance executive. I'll take a table representing large employers, as well as my colleague in the first row who runs one of the largest pharma and medical device companies in the world. I see a patient advocate. My colleague next to me will represent medical schools and pair up with that medical student on the first aisle. There's an information technology and tech entrepreneur in the back, and we are honored to have the CEO of one of the largest electronic medical record (EMR)companies with us.

---

*Fictional

"Miraculously, fifty people representing the twelve sectors of our fragmented healthcare system. Because they have now been rendered incapable of blaming anyone other than themselves, we should have some interesting discussions in what I would describe as the ultimate breakout session. I suspect that each of you will start with what you see when you look in the mirror, and in four hours or so, that confessional should move to a robust discussion about what transformations can occur that would morph into a disruptive dimension for a dramatically different healthcare."

That was it. No thunder or lightning (not even a blackout today). Just the most bizarre and important breakout session in the history of healthcare in America. What happened next was like a scene from one of those zombie movies popular back in the 2010s with creative titles like *Walking Dead, Eat the Living for Lunch,* and *Till Death Do Us Start*. Everyone got up, spontaneously, created small groups by moving their chairs. No confusion, no questioning, no "could you repeat the rules?" It was like everyone involved in this had done this every day of their lives. The vapor strikes again!

Where did we—your humble reporters, authors, contributors— end up? Two of us ended up in tables next to each other—I with the medical school dean (which is where I met the two awesome medical students who also contributed to this undertaking), he with the woman who seemed to be arranging all of this, the woman who seemed to be a walking treasure trove of interesting quotes and who served as the instigator of this morning's exercise. The journalist ended up at the table led by the patient advocate. And our technology innovator, not surprisingly, was seated with the CEO of the EMR company. Twelve tables, twelve transformative ideas. For all intents and purposes, a jury of our peers overseeing the punishment and sentencing for an old system that had lost its luster and prescribing a rehabilitation of American healthcare into a model for the rest of the world.

CHAPTER 9

Mirror, Mirror on the Wall

The American Healthcare Overhaul

Four hours. And then it was done.

One by one, the tables began to report out, but the level of excitement transcended any scripted breakout scribe session that I had ever experienced. In fact, I noticed for the first time that there were no notes taken, no whiteboards, not even any writing instruments on the table, but inextricably, each table ambassador was able to articulate in the oral equivalent of ten pages or less a cogent argument for a transformation that was philosophical, practical, and part of a grander plan. In fact, the remainder of this book will be as close as I can come to a chronicling of those momentous report-outs.

As you know by now, if you have been on the planet for the last ten years leading up to 2026, up until this very day there has been no chronicling of these report-outs. After the conference, everyone dispersed. But the Republican and Democratic tickets, almost out of thin air, supported the "new deal" for healthcare.

For the Democrats it was aptly named *The Dramatically Different Democratic Discourse on a New Healthcare for America*. The Republicans went a different route. Their theme was *Reimagine a Republican Revolution in Healthcare, Rather Than Repeal*. Amazingly though, both platforms were eerily similar and almost word for word what you will read as the first chronicle of those sessions right before your eyes in the ensuing pages.

If you have been paying attention, you might challenge me, in that it was reported that all communications and phones and electronic devices were shut off by the blackout and vapor, "So how the heck were you able to chronicle this story with such amazing skill?"

And while my colleagues and I applaud your attention to detail, and appreciate the compliment, the answer is simple and will be revealed at the end of this book.

Back to the proceedings.

The Bostonian professor with the bow tie and the C-suite guru returned to the stage. "Here is how we should proceed, I believe. I would appreciate if each table could have their ambassador get up, tell us who they represent, what they saw when they looked in the mirror, and, in no more than two sentences, set the stage for the transformation that you will describe after lunch. For some of you, I know that it would take more than two sentences just to recite your title, so we will forego that pre-vapor formality."

The professor did not seem to take offense to that, but added, "Speaking on behalf of my table, I think two things: one, the work we have done here will be remembered many years from now, and two, why the heck did it take us so long?"

With that seemingly obvious but incredibly "to the point" introduction, the fun started.

The medical school dean and student got up, with the dean speaking first, "We represent the future of healthcare. The very DNA that will need to be changed in this new system. We cannot continue to create doctors who fit in to the autonomous, competitive, hierarchical world of the past. We need to promote team-enabled healthcare and creation of high-powered teams. We need to select and educate a new breed of creative, passionate, and flexible physicians." The student, clearly not autonomous, competitive, hierarchical, or afraid, interrupted, "And the accrediting bodies and establishment need to get over their obsession with multiple-choice tests and fragmented episodic education and work toward a continuum of healthcare education that embraces not only the science, but the business and social aspects of healthcare with a heavy dose of cultural diversity and compassion. This way we will have a physician workforce that selects and educates physicians and other healthcare professionals who embrace change, advance an academic and entrepreneurial model, and can be leaders as opposed to followers of healthcare transformation. So the theme for our post-lunch transformation will be 'Creating the **Marcus Welbys*** of the Future,' channeling that icon of compassion and empathy into a post-modern team member in health."

Next came the geek squad, the information technology table. In a very animated fashion, our ambassador of all things futuristic jumped up and started off with a simple statement, "The level of technology used in healthcare today will seem like the dark ages in a few short years. We have to be ready for and embrace that technologic revolution. It needs to start as a blank page. **Michael Dell** said it back in the 2000s, that as you start your journey, 'the first thing you should do is throw away that store-bought map and begin to draw your own.'

"It is great advice for us today as we think about how technology can fundamentally transform how we do things in healthcare. But we have to be creative, bold, *and* accepting of new norms. One of the largest causes of surgical mortality in the twentieth century was anesthesiologists confusing the anesthetic gas with the oxygen. The technologic 'marvel' that eliminated a major cause of death was simply creating a new standard where all oxygen has a square adapter into the tank and all gas has a round one. End of problem! A few places today around the country are heralding the technologic marvel of virtual rounds, where family members—wherever they are—can be part of physician and nurse rounds with their loved ones. That technology, though, has existed for years. It was just our willingness to use it. We talk about Google glasses and goggles, but none of that technology matters without real vision."

Pretty articulate for someone who purportedly develops software all day and very important, as you will see, for the new healthcare. Because technology has *always* been disruptive. What has changed is *our* (purveyors of the American health system) willingness to adopt and adapt and work together to utilize it appropriately.

Next up, the senator, a leading moderate Republican (a term used much more often today than perhaps at the time of this conference).

---

* Marcus Welby: *Marcus Welby, M.D.* was an American medical drama television program aired on ABC from 1969 to 1976. It starred Robert Young as an empathetic, hard-working, family physician who seemingly would do anything to heal the mind, body, and soul of his patients.

"Thank you, and first I want to say how honored I am that I have been invited and asked to speak." (Some habits die hard, even post–BNB vapor.)

"My esteemed and talented group looked in the collective mirror and were amazed at what we saw. While we cannot legislate health, we have done little to promote coordination among caregivers, let alone patients, when it comes to the biggest national security threat in our nation—that of obesity, diabetes, and other chronic diseases. We all share the blame for the fact that an average diabetic sees seven different doctors, none of whom talks to each other and, in many cases, acts at cross-purposes. And while we cannot mandate healthy eating, we can legislate transparency so that menus have caloric and nutritional content boldly displayed. I, for one, look forward to a healthcare future where chronic diseases are first prevented and, if they occur, have coordinated, comprehensive care. We have to create a healthcare system with a capital H and lot of C's with coordination of care across patient conditions, services, and settings over time!"

The physician shot up. "If you want to look at one thing that makes no sense—and I say that in the true spirit of looking in the mirror as a surgeon—it is our guild mentality of assuming that all of us are competent and proficient in our technical and teamwork competence. Here's a shocker for those of you outside the profession. *None* of us who are my age or older have had their technical or teamwork competence objectively assessed in the last twenty to thirty years. I get recertified every year based on a multiple-choice test, but as an amateur pilot, I need to have someone assess my technical competence via simulator and in person every two years. There is something way wrong with the fact that you *know* I am competent if you are flying in my plane, but you have to take my word for it if you are under my knife. We need to replace the whole graduate education (see one, do one, teach one) mentality and the 'I know I'm great, just ask me' philosophy that senior physicians either consciously or subconsciously embrace with a concept of competency-based credentialing and procedure rehearsal studios."

Short, surgical, and maybe not so sweet. But certainly to the point, no surgical pun intended. Also a great example of what can be accomplished if we get over ourselves and commit to these logical solutions. Nothing he described couldn't be done with the technology that existed back in 2016.

The report-outs took shape on an old-fashioned whiteboard:

Bow-Tie Prof: What took us so long?

Medical School Dean: We need to promote team-enabled health.

Medical Student: Stop with the multiple-choice tests already! Teach creativity, communication, and change.

Technology Futurist: Bring on the Healthcare Tech Revolution!

CHAPTER 10

Of Consumerism and Community
Centers of Well-Being

The pace was quickening and it was clear that each individual was excited to have a chance to talk about this optimistic future. The airline CEO could hardly contain herself. She bounded up to the stage next and said, "Look, what I realized is that healthcare needs to be a team sport. The only way we can really make a difference is if employers, providers, and insurers work together to redesign and reengineer care processes to provide better care at a lower cost, using principles that have transformed other industries. Simply put, by thinking of the problem in terms of the system of stakeholders, we can unhinge ourselves from the current deadlocked, pessimistic, and frustrating conversation about healthcare that existed prior to this meeting."

Next up was the MD, MBA, MPH doc. I described him earlier as the population health expert, but because he had more initials than any of us, I thought this might be a more accurate description, as it seemed like we would all be in the population health business in the new healthcare. "First of all, I want to thank my friend and colleague, our first table presenter. He was the dean of my medical college and has been a leader in enhancing traditional medical education. The fact that he has seen the light (or inhaled the vapor) was really enlightening to hear. But we need to go further because, while important, changing the DNA of healthcare one medical student at a time is a slow process—sort of like evolutionary biology—and the only way to speed it up is to mutate our current provider pool, most of whom do not realize they need fundamental change. I gave a course on leadership, followership, and population health for a group of prominent community physicians, and there

53

were two things I heard that made me realize how far we have to go. One of the doc's first reaction was, 'I wasn't born to follow,' and another, during a case study on accountable care organizations, reminded me in a very serious and somber tone that the genius of American medicine is our focus on the individual. He was proud that he viewed the world one patient at a time; he was equally proud that made him a poor allocator of resources. During my report-out, we can discuss what leadership skills will be necessary in the new healthcare, who we need to inject with this knowledge first, and what new jobs and leaders will emerge in different health professions."

That dichotomy of personalizing medicine to the point of the individual gene at the same time that we are thinking broadly in terms of populations seems like it will be a recurring theme. And the cost of personalized medicine, as well as the efficiencies of population health, have been on the minds of insurers since Obamacare was launched, so it was only fitting that the next person to address the group was the CEO of one of the largest payor groups in the country.

"Even before the vapor hit, I could have looked in the mirror and recognized that if all I did was act as a middleman between the patient and provider, then we have no reason to exist. What we are capable of and what hit me like a thunderbolt after the blackout, is our need to partner with providers and patients and employers in any way possible and share what we do best, which is store, analyze, and act on data. Even before I came here, we had one project with a large academic medical center and a sports predictive modeling entity to see if we could leverage our data, the provider's clinical knowledge, and the analytics experts' math and predictive modeling expertise. Rather than hiding our inefficiencies, or negotiating around a failed model, how can we develop creative partnerships both within and outside the healthcare industry together to provide higher-quality care at a lower cost in a way that is much more transparent to patients and employers? That needs to be the question that I wake up every morning trying to answer."

"OK, so now I'm into the true confessions spirit! We have run our hospitals like little fiefdoms waiting for patients to come in, charging them whatever we can get away with, and recognizing that a third party is paying the bill. If we were truly in the hospitality business, we would all be bankrupt." It was the health system CEO's opportunity to describe his newfound approach. "If someone came to my market, a **Steve Jobs** type, and decided to disrupt how we handle our patients, we would lose 80 percent of our patient volume. Instead of treating them like *diseases* or organs, we need to act as if they are *consumers* who have a choice, and turn our hospitals into community centers of well-being. Whoever figures that out will corner the market and make it impossible for others of us to survive without that same consumer and patient-centric mentality. The myth that concierge service is too expensive is just that: a myth. As a hospital CEO, I will need to move from a Blockbuster model (come to my store and I'll get you what you need) to a Netflix model (we are here for you wherever you are). That means I will need to invest in tele-health and other modalities that get my brand to the patient instead of waiting for her to get to me. I have been hanging onto an unsustainable model, and I could not be more excited about using my skills to provide ways to get our care out to where patients are and provide a comfortable venue if they need our hospital services."

An investor-owned insurance CEO and a large health system CEO in basic agreement. The day keeps getting better and better. So just as the dilemma of personalized medicine and population health needs to and can be resolved with creative collaborative thinking, the equally thorny issue of providing community care to individuals wherever they are is not out of reach. The fact that the insurance CEO is often beholden to investors and the health system CEO has much invested in their bricks-and-mortar will clearly need to be resolved.

And just as I was contemplating how that major disruption might play out, the CEO of one of the world's largest pharma companies began. "Not unlike the insurance executive we just heard from, I need to move from selling medical devices and specialty pharmaceuticals to being part of the *solution* team. If my products, data, and expertise can help our customers (who are both patients and providers) provide or take advantage of better care at a lower cost, that will be good for healthcare and good for business. Between us and the large pharmacy providers, such as my friend over in the third row who oversees the largest pharmacy chain in America, we know more about the patient than her provider or hospital does. By the way, truth be told, I didn't need the vapor and blackout to convince me. I was already realizing that if I am just selling commodities, someone will undercut me."

"Riddle me this: Why can I be sitting in my home the day after Thanksgiving watching *Game of Thrones* in my pajamas and do *all* of my holiday shopping, but if I have a stomach ache or a health problem, I can't quickly access a physician or nurse?" The patient advocate continued, "Even the pharmacy chains have figured it out, it's all about *real* patient service. And my aha moment, post-vapor and blackout, is that a good deal of it is our fault. Yes, us, the patients and consumers. Because we complain about everything in every other aspect of our life, but for fifty years we have tolerated and even promoted lousy service from the healthcare and hospital industry. There was a great series called *Through the Patient's Eyes*, which recorded the patient's view of what happens in the hospital. We should play that for every physician and hospital CEO to see if that is how *they* would like to spend their time in the hospital. You as an industry have abandoned all of us during the consumer revolution. How come any of us can do really cool things in every area of our life: holiday shopping on your iPhone or Android, arranging travel through a variety of e-apps, but we still have to access the healthcare system like we did in the 1990s?"

Why consumerism has eluded healthcare is one of those riddles that is difficult to solve. She is right, though. Why the same person who will complain in a restaurant if the food isn't perfect tolerates inedible food and mediocre service at a nightly rate that would embarrass a FOUR SEASONS reservation agent is even more of a mystery.

Then two people got up in unison. I recognized one as the nurse practitioner I had talked to during breakfast; the other was someone I had not met before. "Let's talk about teams . . . and let's all look in the mirror and realize we don't individually have all the answers, but that we can learn from each other." The second individual spoke up, "I have spent my career, first as a chiropractor and then as a DC-MD, questioning treatments that don't work. In any other industry, that desire for new products and treatments would be viewed positively. In healthcare, that makes me an outcast. An outcast with a huge patient population I might add, because *patients* get it. When their physician is too sure of himself but a patient is still not getting control of her chronic disease, when a specialist assumes that the way it is done in other countries must be inferior, and when vitamins and nutrition are virtually ignored in education and research, we are losing great tools in working together toward a healthier community." The nurse interrupted, "So, later this afternoon, we will have three things to talk about as we think about healthcare transformation. Getting serious about creating zero defect units as opposed to just reducing medical errors, viewing non-physician providers as partners instead of subordinates (some state medical societies are still trying to get Doctors of Nursing Practice to not call themselves doctors!), and a model of global health that includes traditional American medicine, nutrition, vitamins, and global solutions."

"Well, I guess I'm the last act." This is one everyone was interested in hearing. The CEO of the world's largest EMR company continued. "Electronic medical records represent the epitome of what is *wrong* and what could be *right* about American healthcare. The promise was great, but at first physicians didn't understand EMRs or their value, and then it was too late. We had created legacy systems that provided electronic representations of paper records but, by and large, did not provide decision support, were not interoperable, and, in many cases, actually decreased the patient–physician relationship and interaction. Oh, and did I mention the price tag. So, the question becomes, at a time of decreasing reimbursement and increased pressure on physician salaries, what is the return on investment on a $200 or $300 million non-customized system? Yes, that's a rhetorical question. I'm proud of what our company has done, but there is so much more we could and should do. Our team will talk about moving from electronic medical records to patient-owned electronic health records. It's one of those many things we've talked about that makes way too much sense to not happen."

✦ ✦ ✦

So now you know how the healthcare you enjoy today came into being back in 2016. Mystery solved. That's how it all happened. The rest of this book will chronicle exactly what was developed as strategies to reimagine healthcare in America. The combined knowledge and insights of the "vaporized" invitees to the conference became the ambassadors for the revolution. The broad strategies highlighted on the next pages became a virtual field manual for an optimistic future in healthcare (almost as if an alien had kidnapped us and given us the answers). In this case, the answer was right on the tip of our tongues, and all it took was some introspection to loosen it into consciousness. Many of these ideas will seem obvious to you now that healthcare has embraced them, but imagine if you were reading this for the first time in 2016.

Oh, and by the way, while it's not a mystery what happened to healthcare in the past ten years after THE EVENT, there are still some mysteries about those two days and our involvement. But those answers will need to wait until the last chapter.

Enjoy the disruptive dozen . . . and I'll be back with you before long!

CHAPTER 11

Of Wizards, Mindsets, and
Perinatal Mortality

So, how do we develop these disruptors?" asked the information technology professional. "It's not like some alien is going to abduct us and send us back ten years later with a Wharton professor to guide us." (See *The Phantom Stethoscope: A Field Manual for Finding an Optimistic Future in Medicine*.)

"No, of course not." A new participant appeared—tall, lanky, bearded, and looking every bit his 150 years of age. I blinked, but no matter how many times I blinked it looked like . . . a wizard, hair, beard, robe. Aliens, wizards, who organized this conference? "The only way you will truly transform the system is to go out there and see what is really going on with the no-blame transformative mindset you currently possess. I am sent here to help you do that."

"OK, so we are just going to have all of us traipse through hospitals, insurers, pharma companies and go unnoticed. Sounds like a great plan!" exclaimed a very frustrated physician.

"Actually, that is exactly what you are going to do. I will make you invisible so that you can investigate with your new mindset what is really going on out there. I believe the 'new eyes' that the blackout has afforded you will add some discomfort that will have you question some of the 'truths' that you held to be self-evident and will lead you to some very different conclusions as well as help you develop the dozen disruptors that you seek to find."

"I don't mean to be disrespectful, but this is not exactly a Hobbit battle in Middle Earth," was the response. The wizard gave a wizened smile (the only kind he knows how to give, apparently), "Actually, as

J. R. R. Tolkien said in that famous book," he laughed, "the board is set and the pieces are moving. We come to it at last, the great battle of our time. In your case, the battle for the soul of healthcare in America. The resources America has committed to healthcare and training is unparalleled. There is nothing comparable to the 141 academic medical centers in the United States. But for all that, you are #17 in the world in key healthcare indicators.

"So join me, you will be invisible, and the first place you will go is the epicenter of the new healthcare," the wizard continued.

"Are we going to Boston?" the surgeon from Massachusetts General Hospital (MGH) asked with a straight face.

"No, I was speaking metaphorically. If we are going to fundamentally change healthcare, we have to start with the trainees—the students and residents who will represent the new providers in the transformation. So, we are going to an academic medical center, and we will look at the selection and education of students, as well as the mindset and training of resident physicians."

"Well, good luck getting through the traffic this time of day," said the nurse practitioner.

"I have a feeling that a wizard will have a slightly more sophisticated way of getting our invisible butts across town," the pharma CEO calmly stated.

CHAPTER 12

See One, Do One, Teach One.
No More

If you want to look at one thing that makes no sense—and I say that in the true spirit of looking in the mirror as a surgeon—it is our guild mentality of assuming that all of us are proficient in our technical and teamwork competence. Here's a shocker for those of you outside the profession. None of us who are my age or older have had their technical or teamwork competence objectively assessed in the last twenty to thirty years. I get recertified every year based on a multiple-choice test, but as an amateur pilot, I need to have someone assess my technical competence by simulation and in person every two years. There is something way wrong with the fact that you know I am competent if you are flying in my plane, but you have to take my word for it if you are under my knife. We need to replace the whole graduate education (see one, do one, teach one) mentality and the "I know I'm great, just ask me" philosophy of senior physicians with a concept of competency-based credentialing and procedure rehearsal studios.

And so it was. In the blink of an eye, literally, the group was transported to a delivery room where a premature baby had just been delivered. "Have you ever intubated a premature baby?" the resident was asked by the pediatrician. No, I have only observed. "Good, there's a first time for everything. Remember see one, do one, teach one." And so, a procedure that requires intense fine motor coordination—namely, finding the trachea and identifying the appropriate airway in a baby weighing less than two pounds—was performed by the resident on a *real* baby.

After the procedure, the attending physician walked out to the delivery lounge, the invisible wizard waved a wand, and the attending physician looked confused, and then started a soliloquy that led to one of the disruptors.

"Actually this makes no sense," the attending physician began, looking at the invisible wizard but, in essence, speaking to himself. "When any of us travel on an airplane, we *know* the pilot is competent, because within the last year that individual has had his/her technical competence assessed and if he/she did not fall within a narrow mean and standard deviation, he/she is not flying your plane. Even beyond technical competence, many of the crises that have been averted in aviation, such as the successful landing of US Air 1549 in the Hudson River were based on teamwork concepts learned in crew resource management training sessions—in essence, simulated opportunities for the entire team to "practice" emergency skills together while passengers' lives are not at risk."

"If we are going to move from thinking about healthcare *reform* to creating healthcare *transformation*, the most striking example of where healthcare has fallen behind other high-reliability organizations is in our ability to assess and certify technical and teamwork competence. When I think about it, if I were a pilot I would have to get my technical competence *objectively* assessed every year, but as an obstetrician, the last time anyone objectively assessed my technical skills was in 1984. I get recertified by filling out a multiple-choice test every year. So, the level of confidence that my patients have that I could perform minimally invasive surgery was that I had the cognitive skills to pass the multiple-choice test and the dexterity to pick up a pencil and not go too far outside the lines.

"Even more striking is the fact that, given an aging surgeon population, we have no way of objectively assessing someone who has an excessive amount of complications. In a survey that we are currently performing around the country, we found that the most common means of dealing with an experienced surgeon who has had excessive surgical complications is that he/she is locally proctored. The obvious fallacy with that approach is the lack of objectivity—usually with the 'proctor' being a colleague or a competitor with all the attendant legal, emotional, and subjective baggage leading to unintended consequences and, in most cases, inaction.

"Most importantly, the entire see one, do one, teach one rubric for teaching surgeons and other providers is both anachronistic and dangerous—especially for the *person* on the other side of the table. It often takes decades to get a new drug approved in this country because we want to ensure that no patient is harmed before the drug has been exhaustively tested. Similarly, new medical devices take years to win approval with the same conservative "do no harm" mentality by the FOOD AND DRUG ADMINISTRATION (FDA) regulators. However, once a new device is approved, all bets are off as to ensuring that the surgeon *behind* the instrument is as safe as the instrument itself. Many of us lived through the 'learning curve' days of early minimally invasive surgery when procedures such as cholecystectomy or robotic surgery were proved 'safe' by a cadre of early pioneers, with almost no objective way of teaching or accrediting the next wave of those that want to perform the procedure. What we take as a given—that healthcare will be more inefficient and that patients will suffer more morbidity during these learning phases—will be even more inexcusable in a value-based purchasing future in which payors and patients will expect technical and teamwork competence and excellence.

"The best disruptive investment you could make is to defragment the thousands of simulation centers that each hospital possesses and create regional assessment of technical and teamwork institutes or CENTERS FOR ASSESSMENT OF SURGICAL AND TEAMWORK LEARNING AND SIMULATION (CASTLS).

"As an entrepreneurial academic initiative, we could take the millions of dollars that are spent on bureaucracy in specialty societies and work with experts around the world to develop models based on best practices and successful skills acquisition models in other industries. The development of surgical skill requires both qualitative and quantitative technical and clinical experience. With this experience, surgical judgment will generally follow.

"Finally, there is a less-well-defined attitude or surgical mentality that must be possessed or developed. With this mindset, the individual is highly prepared for and focused on the operation, works through barriers and other types of difficulties to ensure a good outcome, and at times will push outside of his/her comfort zone for the benefit of the patient. The ability to develop these skills through mentored simulation centers rather than in the 'heat of the battle' of an operating or delivery room has been shown to increase both surgical competence and confidence. No resident physician in training should be performing any difficult procedure until he/she has proven that he or she has the requisite technical skills and confidence to perform that procedure on an inanimate object.

"Rather than relying solely on the chance encounters during the four years of residency, a simulation curriculum should be based upon structured and stepwise progression. The focus is shifted from patient care to the trainee. Residents do part of their training in an environment where they are no longer expected to step up and perform a perfect operation. This is a much less stressful training environment for both the trainee and faculty and, more importantly, shortens the learning curve toward improved patient care.

"We need to create a groundswell among surgeons, other physicians and healthcare providers, industry, hospitals, and accrediting bodies to fundamentally transform the way we educate and train those of us who perform these highly advanced procedures. If we changed our training in this way, developed these centers, learned from other industries, and had our specialty societies require periodic 'checkups' for every practitioner around technical and teamwork competence, the see one, do one, teach one mentality will be an historic footnote alongside blood-letting and frontal lobotomies.

"The simple fact is that healthcare is alone as a high-reliability organization (HRO) that does not mandate periodic assurance of technical and teamwork competence.* Teamwork and the ability to prove participation in a high-powered team is a non-negotiable aspect of the training of all HROs *except* for healthcare.

"One of the advantages of requiring periodic simulated assessment for all physicians as it relates to their technical and teamwork competence is the potential for immediate feedback, which is obviously much more difficult in the middle of a real procedure with a human patient. Immediate feedback is also a characteristic of effective team performance. Team members must monitor each other and provide each other feedback to maximize team functioning. To ensure that feedback occurs, team members must be trained to deliver timely, behavioral, and specific feedback to one another. The ability to monitor each other's performance and effectively provide feedback to other team members is a critical facet of achieving higher reliability in healthcare and elsewhere.

"We need to look at healthcare errors and training as similar to the aviation crises that triggered crew resource management in the 1970s, when aviation safety experts recognized that many of the disasters occurred not because of technical skill deficiencies, but because of communication and lack of teamwork coordination. It is concerned with the cognitive and interpersonal skills needed to manage resources within an organized system, not so much with the technical knowledge and skills required to operate equipment. In this context, cognitive skills are defined as the mental processes used for gaining and maintaining situational awareness, for solving problems, and for making decisions—all crucial in split-second decisions in healthcare and only a minor part of most graduate medical education training curricula. In many opera-

---

* HROs: those organizations that function in hazardous, fast-paced, and highly complex technological systems, essentially error-free for long periods of time. Roberts and Rousseau identified eight characteristics of HROs: (1) hyper-complexity, (2) tightly coupled, (3) extreme hierarchical differentiation, (4) many decision makers working in complex communication networks, (5) high degree of accountability, (6) frequent, immediate feedback regarding decisions, (7) compressed time factors, and (8) synchronized outcomes (Roberts, Karlene H. and Denise M. Rousseau. 1989. Research in Nearly Failure-Free, High-Reliability Organizations: Having the Bubble. IEEE Transactions on Engineering Management. 36(2): 132–139).

tional systems, as in other walks of life, skill areas often overlap with each other, and as such, the approach in healthcare should include not only the technical knowledge and skills required to operate equipment or perform specific operations, but also the cognitive and interpersonal skills needed to effectively manage a team-based, high-risk activity such as surgery or the delivery of a high-risk baby."

Yes, we witnessed it. Trancelike, that monologue by that attending physician—who, minutes earlier, had felt comfortable with the old way of training residents—forever changed him and us. That "groundswell" did indeed occur, and today, no resident would be allowed to do any procedure on a living patient before proving his/her competence on a simulator. Today in 2026, if someone asks you "is your surgeon qualified and can they prove it?" your answer can be a confident "yes!" because he or she has had their technical competence objectively assessed within the past few years *and* they are not performing surgery on you unless they have been within a mean and a standard deviation of technical and teamwork competence.

Changes 2016–2026

What's Changed the Most in Competency and Teamwork Assessment and Training in Healthcare in 2026?

1. Every surgeon must have his/her technical and teamwork competence objectively assessed at one of three regional training centers every seven years.

2. If a new technology is developed, the entire surgical team must prove their competence on a simulated model *before* operating on a patient.

3. Any physician who has more than one major complication in a six-month period must be assessed via simulation and prove that he/she is within a mean and standard deviation of the norm.

What Happened in 2016 That Led to the Transformation?

1. Millennials wanted proof that their surgeon was competent to perform the procedure that they were contemplating. The "Is Your Surgeon Qualified and Can They Prove It" campaign was born.

2. Medical device companies partnered with simulation centers to include non-human training in the technical and teamwork aspects of the new procedure into the price of buying the new technology.

3. Residents and medical trainees were prohibited to perform any procedure on a human until they had proven competence and proficiency on an inanimate object.

CHAPTER 13

From Marcus Welby to House

How Did We Get There?

We cannot continue to create doctors who fit in to the autonomous, competitive, hierarchical world of the past. We need to promote team-enabled healthcare and creation of high-powered teams. We need to select and educate a new breed of creative, passionate, and flexible physicians. [The student, clearly not autonomous, competitive, hierarchical, or afraid, interrupted.] And the accrediting bodies and establishment need to get over their obsession with multiple-choice tests and fragmented episodic education and work toward a continuum of healthcare education that embraces not only the science, but the business and social aspects of healthcare with a heavy dose of cultural diversity and compassion. This way we will have a physician workforce that selects and educates physicians and other healthcare professionals who embrace change, advance an academic and entrepreneurial model, and can be leaders as opposed to followers of healthcare transformation. So the theme for our post-lunch transformation will be "Creating the Marcus Welbys of the Future," channeling that icon of compassion and empathy into a post-modern team member in health. *

A simple touch of the ring and we were hurtling through space to where, another hospital? No, this time we were in a living room in the 1960s.

---

* A medical college selects for empathy: Roscoe, L. A., English, A. & Monroe, A. D. H. (2014). Scholarly excellence, leadership experiences, and collaborative training: Qualitative results from a new curricular initiative. *Journal of Contemporary Medical Education*, 2, 163–167.

How did we know?

Well, for one thing, there was a picture of the New York City World's Fair in a house that looked pretty new. There was a copy of the **Rolling Stones**' first album (yes, in real vinyl) that also looked pretty new. And just in case you are impressed with my deductive skills, there was a newspaper on the table that was dated September 12, 1964.

And on the TV (a nineteen-incher with rabbit ears) was one of the most popular shows on TV, *Marcus Welby, M.D.*

The wizard spoke, "Think about it. TV shows are written by lay people who view the profession as they see it. In the 1960s, the quintessential doctor TV show featured **Marcus Welby**, MD: a primary care physician who made house calls, didn't charge patients who couldn't afford it, maybe even delivered a calf on the side of the road as he was coming home to lunch—all before performing difficult surgery on a young patient as the climax of the episode. To people outside the profession, doctors were empathetic, all-knowing 'gods' who could do no wrong as long as they had an understanding smile and a black bag."

There was a little twitch, and there we were in a similar living room fifty years later. How did I know? You guessed it—the newspaper read September 12, 2014. On the much bigger, clearer TV was a rerun from one of the most popular TV shows of the beginning of the twenty-first century, *House, M.D.**

So, these same individuals outside the profession no longer viewed us as all-knowing empathetic gods; we were now drug-addicted, narcissistic (admittedly brilliant beyond words), twenty-first-century physicians.

The wizard again, "So how did physicians go from saints to sinners so quickly in the public's eye? Solving that question does not take a magical ring or a wise old man of 150 years of age. Why do physicians resist change rather than lead transformation? How would we need to

---

*Marcus Welby and House: Marcus Welby, previously footnoted. *House, M.D.* was an American medical drama television program aired on Fox from 2004–2012. Dr. House was virtually the opposite of Dr. Welby and was portrayed by Hugh Laurie as a narcissistic, drug-addicted genius diagnostician.

change the way we select and educate physicians to turn us back from Dr. Houses to Dr. Welbys?"

I had a strange feeling the answer was not going to be simple, and it required a bit of time travel again. This time we were not in a living room watching TV, but in a medical school admissions committee in 2026.

How did I know it was a medical school admissions committee? Because there was a hologram with a very deanly looking individual addressing the group saying, "Welcome to the interviewing session for the medical school class of 2031." (Apparently medical school was now only three years.) Also, because that same hologram had scrolling under it (yes, hologram apps had adopted the same annoying technology of CNN and other news shows in the 2010s):

President Jenna Bush will be debating Democratic nominee **Chelsea Clinton** in a tight race for the 2028 presidential race.

Harrison Ford has signed on for one last Indiana Jones sequel tentatively titled, Indiana Jones: The Legend of Bingo Night.

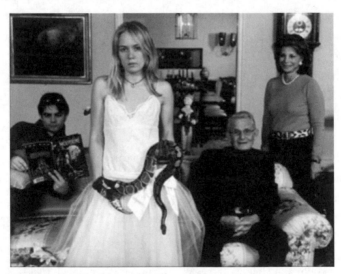

What's going on in this picture?
Tina Barney: Family Commission with Snake. 2010. **Tina Barney** *is an American-born photographer best known for her large-scale color portraits of family and friends.*

But stranger than any of those was the fact that these applicants were not being interviewed in a windowless hospital room, but were standing in a beautiful art museum. Up on the wall was this picture.

The wizard appeared in hologram fashion next to the dean, and while we were invisible, he apparently was able to be seen by the admissions committee.

"**Dean Wurmer**, pardon me, but before you start your interviews, I have a group of guests who are both invisible and would take too long to explain what they are doing here. To my guests from 2016, Dean Wurmer will be able to hear any questions you have but will not be able to see you. Dean, they are very interested in what looks like a far cry from the medical school—look to the left of you, look to the right of you, one of you will get accepted—admissions of the past. Could you explain what's changed and why?"

Apparently the holographic dean as well as the physical members of the admissions committee did not think any of this strange.

The dean continued.

"Back in 2016, we were training physicians of the past. And if you asked anybody back in 2016 why they can't fundamentally change the way we select or educate physicians, they would say they couldn't fundamentally change selection criteria or educational curricula because of *US News and World Report* (USNWR) rankings, or the AMERICAN ASSOCIATION OF MEDICAL COLLEGE accreditation, or because of their curriculum committee. They blamed everyone but themselves."

"Wow, that seems to be a common theme even outside our little vapor-induced conclave," said the invisible nurse practitioner.

"In fact, back in 2016, I gave a talk for USNWR on the hospitals of tomorrow," the dean continued, "and the editor introduced me and I got up there, thanked him, and said 'I'll probably never get invited back here, but you're part of the problem, because if I really start to select and educate emotionally intelligent students not based on science GPA, MCATs, and organic chemistry grades, I'll go down ten points in your rankings.' And I gave what I thought was a very compelling speech with good data about the kind of physicians we would need for ten years from now, based on self-awareness and empathy. At the end of the speech, the editor got up there and said, 'You know, you're right.' I said, 'I am?' He said, 'You're right you'll never get invited back here,' and I never was."*

Fortunately, we have come a long way and recognized that it is now all about team-enabled healthcare. Whereas most ranking systems until 2020 were based on research funding, reputation of the past, and all those other parameters that made for *House, M.D.*, the doctors we needed for the future (and the healers most people would want to care for them) are those who can deliver team-enabled care, doctors working closely with multidisciplinary, care-delivery teams.

"Yes, but the reason for those admission criteria have always been that if I know nineteen reasons you have a headache and someone else can only memorize fifteen, then I am a better diagnostician because he/she may miss four reasons," said the neurosurgeon to his invisible colleagues.

"You might say that memorization was crucial because if someone could recite an organic chemistry formula, he or she can store more possibilities for a differential diagnosis in his or her brain," the dean clarified.

"My point exactly," exclaimed the neurosurgeon to no one in particular.

"A sort of epiphany happened in 2018 when three events conspired to change all that," the dean explained.

"First of all, as deans of medical colleges became younger and more savvy, they rebelled against the ranking systems of the past. Ninety of the one hundred forty medical schools refused to put their data into the USNWR database. At the same time, genomics and other medical knowledge grew so fast that no human brain on the planet could memorize everything they needed to know. Finally, APPLE acquired IBM and created a Watson clone (that looms holographically in a form that looks suspiciously like **Steve Jobs**), which can memorize every genetic sequence and all medical knowledge, so that the *only* function physicians

---

*Medical students don't get organization communication and teamwork skills: "What Skills Should New Internal Medicine Interns Have in July? A National Survey of Internal Medicine Residency Program Directors," *Academic Medicine*, vol. 89, issue 3 (March 2014), 432–435.

serve is to add the human aspects to this computerized brain—those very same human aspects that were not selected for and certainly not cultivated in 2016 medical school admissions.

"So its not surprising that, back in 2016, given the way we selected and educated physicians, after four years of medical school and three to seven years of graduate medical education, the young physician often begins his or her studies as an idealistic, optimistic overachiever, but by the end of the process, often loses those endearing qualities," surmised the primary care physician.

"Yes, I think educators of your era euphemistically called it 'the hidden curriculum,'" the 2026 dean agreed. "Between your selection process and the fact that much of your students' clinical clerkships were overseen by physicians not willing to change, those young, idealistic, even creative young trainees took on much of the jaded, pessimistic, House-like qualities of their mentors.

"I spent much of my career investigating why business leaders get so excited about changes in healthcare and why those of us physicians who actually have to live with and implement the change dread it. The answer came to me in a rather simple experiment called The Pheasant Egg Auction, in which a professor from the WHARTON SCHOOL OF BUSINESS and I compared physicians and MBAs from around the country. In a case study format, we challenged the participants to solve a problem that required collaboration, creativity, and navigating ambiguity. The bottom line is that 82 percent of the MBAs got to the 'everybody wins' scenario and only 11 percent of the docs were able to find a solution. Through this and other studies, we theorized that the way we select and educate physicians has created a cult around four biases: competitive, autonomous, hierarchical, and noncreative.

"In our 'experiment,' physicians seemed hesitant to risk cooperation, fearing a win/lose result that might make them look bad. In fact, doctors sometimes expressed the feeling that they would rather have everyone lose than give anyone else a chance to get more than his or her fair share. The autonomy bias is even a greater risk for a future in which more and more physicians find themselves in large organizations. Clinical practice often demands that physicians act autonomously, and medical selection and training emphasized that need. However, the more complex that medical practice became, the more autonomy became a liability by limiting opportunities for creative partnerships. How many times are medical students told that there is a "pecking order" in medicine? While this hierarchy is necessary in some research and clinical arenas, in which unambiguous relationships and rapid response to orders means the difference between life and death, it is a significant liability in a health transformation environment that increasingly calls for working partnerships and 'teams' with a variety of players in the healthcare arena.

"So, no wonder, in a survey we completed back in your time, in 2014, 70 percent of physicians practicing three years or less felt insecure about the future of medicine. Simply put, they felt that they had learned half of what they needed to know. They learned microbiology and biochemistry, cardiology, and surgery. But they didn't learn how to manage change, effectively communicate, be an individual in an organization, be a leader (or a follower for that matter), make patients happy, run an effective meeting, or market themselves or their practice.

"Even back thirty years ago," he concluded, "the INSTITUTE OF MEDICINE in its monograph on the "Quality of Healthcare in America" stated that the 'American healthcare delivery system is in need of fundamental change. Trying harder will not work. Changing systems of care will.' It is clear that the selection and education mechanisms that we have employed in our training of physicians in the last fifty years required a similar transformation."

"I get the autonomy, hierarchy, and competitive thing—but noncreative? Physicians are some of the most creative people I know," said the insurance executive.

"You are right, physicians are just as creative as anyone, but much of that creativity gets sucked out of them through the physician training cycle."

"When we asked MBAs for the three most important skills sets responsible for their success, creativity was one of them in 92 percent of the cases. When we asked physicians the same question, creativity only made the top three in 11 percent of responses. So what happened, over the last ten years, as external factors were creating new rules around healthcare? If you *believed* you were creative, you loved that change. The more things swirled around you and the more chaotic they were, the more convinced and committed you were that your creativity skill set would put you in good stead.

"Because physicians were autonomous, competitive, hierarchical professionals who did *not believe* that they could win through creativity or thinking differently, they assumed change was bad for them in their own minds. So entrepreneurs ruled the day, while many physicians fought the inevitable change. That was, of course, until that strange event in 2016 with the blackout thing and the 'Twelve Disruptors of the Future in Healthcare.' That changed everything!"

CHAPTER 14

White Dresses, Black Turtlenecks, and Snakes

Wow they know about us, very cool," said the primary care doc. "This whole lost weekend wasn't a waste after all."

Dean Wurmer, the 2026 dean, explained exactly what had changed in education and the selection of future physicians.

"So, we recognized that the only way to keep medicine and health-care in the hands of humans was to emphasize those qualities that only humans can still do—namely, effective communication, observing vs. seeing, and reading between the lines of human emotions—because the machines will always do a better job of memorizing the Krebs cycle than any human brain ever can.

"We now choose students based on emotional intelligence, self-awareness, and empathy once they have reached a minimum of proficiency in objective, multiple-choice-type science and didactic knowledge. We also segment students so that self-awareness takes a greater role than science GPA for those interested in becoming a practicing physician, while the traditional parameters take on increased importance for those wanting to become physician scientists. It amazes me that, back in your time, you didn't even perform technical simulation diagnostics to steer and select students based on technical skills (or steer them away from those specialties). Now a student is 'guided' into a career choice based on *both* their proclivities as well as their inherent assets and talents.

"By the way, you might notice that our computer hologram colleagues look like **Steve Jobs**. That's because the human Jobs recognized all this back at the turn of the twenty-first century when he said, 'Have the courage to follow your heart and intuition. They somehow know what you truly want to become, everything else is secondary.' He could have been talking about today's young physicians, who now use both sides of their brain—the linear, literal, rational, logical, and lab-oriented along with the intuitive, imaginative, creative, and bedside-oriented. They partner with their computer holographic colleagues who can and do memorize all the medical knowledge known, record all the patient's symptoms, and offer true decision support for their 'human partner.' Now when we talk about team-enabled healthcare, it is the physician, nurse, other human professionals, and all artificial intelligence involved in the patient's care."

"So what I still don't understand is why you are selecting medical students in an art museum," asked the neurosurgeon to himself.

"So you might be wondering why we now use this picture to select medical students," the dean mused.

"I thought they could hear us," the neurosurgeon mused.

"Why don't you just watch," the dean continued.

The first applicant walked in.

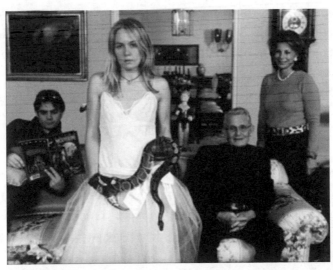

What's going on in this picture?
Tina Barney: Family Commission with Snake. 2010. **Tina Barney** *is an American-born photographer best known for her large-scale color portraits of family and friends.*

"What do you see in this picture?" was the first question asked to the young aspiring medical school applicant.

The applicant immediately chimed in, "I see a woman in a white dress, a man in a turtleneck, and a snake," and immediately described in detail everything he could "see" in the picture.

"OK, but what do you observe in this picture?" the interviewer asked.

"I observe a woman in a white dress, a man in a turtleneck, and a snake," searching for some other detail that he might have missed.

"I understand that is what you see, but what's the picture telling you; what is it emoting to you?" The interviewer gave it one more try.

"It's emoting to me that there's a guy in a black turtleneck, a woman in a white dress, and a snake of some kind." The applicant seemed increasingly frustrated that he must have missed something.

"Thank you very much. We will be in touch," concluded the admissions officer, and the prospective student was dismissed.

The second applicant, a young woman walked in.

Same question: "What do you see in this picture?"

She did not answer right away, but when she did, she answered confidently, "I believe the snake represents the relationship between the woman and her family. I believe that the woman in the white dress is feeling increasingly disenfranchised, perhaps on the eve of her wedding day and . . ."

"Excellent answer," the interviewer retorted. "It is clear that you can not just see, but observe. We will *definitely* be back in touch with you."

"I'm not sure I quite understand why that matters," said the neurosurgeon, again seemingly to himself.

"Why does that matter?" continued the dean. "It matters because even today, as an obstetrician having delivered over a thousand babies, I recognize a simple fact that the admissions committees of your time neglected to realize. It is fairly easy delivering an eight-pound healthy baby to a healthy parent.

"It's not easy (even though it almost never happens in 2026 with predictive genomic testing) delivering an unscheduled baby with Downs syndrome or another congenital anomaly.

"The first question the patient always asks in that case is, 'What does this mean, doctor?'

"I've watched very smart obstetricians like the first lad who stood before the admissions committee immediately discuss the chromosomal anomaly or the medical complications they had memorized attendant to that diagnosis.

The second applicant, that young lady who we will undoubtedly accept, would marshal her self-awareness and empathy and recognize immediately that 'what does it mean?' has nothing to do with chromosomes or medical complications, but rather the patient and her partner wanting to emotionally understand what it means to their image of a perfect baby. *Her* response would be one that recognizes the emotional nature of the question and she would say something like this:

" 'I believe what you're asking me is what this means to your image of a perfect baby. This baby has some issues that we had not expected, but she is a beautiful baby. We will be with you and communicate with you over the next several days, and most importantly I will get you in touch with some other families who have gone through the same experience.'

"That thirty seconds is *the* difference in how that couple reacts to the set of circumstances and in how they perceive and bond with their new baby.

"Think about it. The Watson*-APPLE hologram would be able to best memorize the genomics and potential complications. The *only* value the human physician adds in this era is our ability to understand the human and emotional component of the unexpected outcome. That is why we now select applicants in a very different way."

"So, is there any science to how this is done, or is it just a day at the art museum?" asked the pharma executive, clearly having played rounds of golf with enough physicians to be cynical about the growing trend in holism in medical education.

"Actually, the data was quite evident even back in 2016. At HARVARD, a study was done in 2010 that medical and dental students who took a

---

*Watson: a question-answering augmented intelligence computer system able to answer questions in natural language, developed by IBM. Without changes in the education and selection of future doctors, it will make us irrelevant.

semester-long art course made 40 percent more observations based on medical images, and their observations were significantly more sophisticated. At UNIVERSITY OF TEXAS, SAN ANTONIO, even earlier, a study was done in which they took interdisciplinary students—medicine, nursing, physical therapy—and even in a few four-hour sessions, they demonstrated increased observation skills and were able to utilize skill sets leading to better teamwork. At the University of South Florida, a course in art included public health students, who consistently were able to see outside of the frame of a work of art to assess social and environmental influences. In other words, it has been clear for a while that the ability to 'observe as opposed to see' and the self-awareness of 'reading or hearing between the lines' when communicating with a patient is a learned skill not significantly different from technical skill sets learned throughout medical school and residency."

"You made a big deal about choosing physicians of the future through your very different interview process. How do you maintain that focus in the new curriculum?" the invisible but audible primary care doc asked.

"Good question. We do, as you suggest, actively search for emotional intelligence characteristics of students—self-awareness, empathy, and the ability to be a change catalyst—that make it most likely for them to be successful in a leadership role. We then want to make sure that we have a futuristic curriculum that emphasizes leadership education, values and ethics, disparities, and health systems and policy so our students can become leaders as opposed to followers of healthcare transformation.

"We have also totally changed our curriculum in both undergraduate pre-med programs as well as medical and nursing schools. In undergraduate programs, we concentrate more on anthropology and other human factors along with the science prerequisites and no longer screen pre-med students based on ability to memorize complicated organic chemistry formulas. MCATs are optional and usually reserved for those students who were not able to prove their ability to grasp scientific knowledge during their undergraduate program.

In medical school, it would seem ludicrous to do what you did in 2016. The concept of taking energetic students who have just spent four years in a classroom—whether real, online, or holographic—and then subject them to another two years in a classroom would be unthinkable today. Almost the entire first two years of medical school in 2026 is taught in parallel with simulated and augmented intelligence patient skills.

So, microbiology, biochemistry, and anatomy are taught through various online and other modalities, partly because we recognized something that was known even at your time. The generation you used to call Millennials did not show up to class because the old way of having a professor interact with students was already antiquated and ineffective back in 2016. I remember as a young faculty member back in 2016 that the class would be full the first day, but unless the professor was exceptionally talented and/or entertaining, anyone who did show up to class was pretty lonely after that.

"We now concentrate on items that require human professors—health systems competencies, cultural competencies, leadership competencies, eliminating health disparities, and understanding a student's own biases. Every medical student takes a minor, a college within a college; some of the most popular are design, disparities, business and entrepreneurship, research techniques, teaching skills, global health, engineering, law, medical humanities, medical writing, and even music theory.

"These minors earned in the college within a college differentiate each student and often become specialized areas of interest that the student-turned-practitioner maintains throughout his or her career. By the way, almost none of this is school-centric. By that I mean that all courses and minors are totally intermixed among nursing, medicine, and the other health professions. Inter-professional learning is no longer an eccentricity or something we write articles about. It is built into the DNA of our students. One of the most valuable aspects of the new curriculum is a summer internship between years one and two in which students follow and interact with a leader of their choosing. This may be an entrepreneur, the state's surgeon general, a health network medical officer, or even an artist, journalist, or public health worker in another country.

"All of this is to alter the old 'captain of the ship' mentality that worked well in the twentieth century and is now replaced by a 'key member of the team' philosophy that, in most clinical situations, includes doctors, nurses, clinical pharmacists, physical therapists, nutritionists, mental health professionals, augmented intelligence robots, and other members of both the human and the artificial intelligence team."

"I noticed you used the AI word as 'augmented intelligence.' Don't you mean artificial intelligence?" the IT guru asked, sensing he knew something that could add to the conversation.

"No, not at all," the dean smiled knowingly. "We recognized early on that our 'emotional' intelligence and the robot's super brain are different. In fact, in health professional schools, such as medical school, we now concentrate more on the human elements. In fact, every student has an academic coach and a personal mentor. While a mentor/mentee connection is open-ended and can span decades, the more formal coaching relationship is used to address specific issues; after a particular challenge has been addressed, the relationship moves to an as-needed basis. In 2019, we even instituted peer mentors (another student paired to you) who, along with your personal mentor, helps the student overcome any gaps in leadership or biases that were identified during the 360-degree interview process. He/she performs the same function for his/her peer.

"Your entire fourth year of medical school is geared toward getting you ready for your chosen field—technical skills for surgical specialties, research skills for those going into discovery fields, entrepreneurship and MBA skills for those choosing business tracks, and public health skills for those choosing a career in lessening health disparities. We now have 25 percent of students who never take a residency because they are entering entrepreneurial, population health, information technology, or other fields in which their medical degree is crucial but whereby they have chosen not to practice. Those who do practice have overcome the education and selection biases that plagued the early part of the twenty-first century."

The 2016 medical school dean, sounding exasperated, stated, "What's amazing about this is that none of this is new information. We knew it all along and chose to ignore the data. In essence, while the world around us was changing, we continued to select and educate medical students with only incremental changes over fifty years. It shouldn't have taken an abnormal event like the vapor to force us into this epiphany. For God's sake, the JOSIAH MACY JR. FOUNDATION report, in the 2000s, made exactly that point when it stated that, "Medical education has not kept pace with the growing demands of an increasingly complex healthcare system. Medical students too often graduate without the knowledge and skills that twenty-first-century physicians need and without fully appreciating the role that professional values, leadership competencies, and attitudes play."

Dean Wurmer smiled and seemed to address the invisible dean. "I understand that this day started with a wizard talking about how people from outside the profession view us, from **Marcus Welby** to **House**! As medical school deans, we can both appreciate that we don't have much time to watch TV. Of course, in 2026, there is an implantable AMAZON and NETFLIX (ALL-FLIX) chip in our brain, so all we have to do is ask to see any program and it shows up as a holographic image. Now, our doctor TV shows are all about the interactions between the humans and augmented intelligence robots and the seemingly funny situations that occur between the human and artificial intelligence brains.

"But as one of those who is getting older and will eventually slow down and most likely become a consumer of healthcare services, I am hopeful that my future physicians will be empathetic, holistic, creative, and caring. That while they may not be able to memorize the Krebs cycle, they will have enough scientific knowledge base to interpret the data from their robot counterparts but, more importantly, have the emotional intelligence to know when to consult their iPhone XX. I want my physician to recognize his or her limitations and know when and whom to go to for the appropriate information that will best help them develop a plan for my care and communicate it to me.

"And yes," he concluded with a wry smile. "I hope that the personality of Dr. House as a model of physician behavior becomes as dated as Dr. Welby might seem to you in 2016!"

Changes 2016–2026

What's Changed the Most in Selection and Education of Physicians for the Future in 2026?

1. Objective criteria, such as science GPA, are used to establish minimums for admission. After that, those results, as well as the school you attended, etc., are blinded, and students are chosen based on communication, empathy, and other "human" skills.

2. Medical schools are specialized to a greater degree, and the selection and curriculum are quite different. Therefore, a research intensive–dominant school will look at objective science and research parameters more traditionally, and its curriculum more resembles a traditional one. A clinical practitioner–dominant school will admit based on self-awareness and empathy with less reliance on traditional parameters. An entrepreneurial-innovation–dominant school will select and educate based on creativity and proven ability to "think different."

3. Institutes of emerging health professions house the most sought-after majors among undergraduates. The majors are developed by the students themselves with assistance from their instructor/mentors.

What Happened in 2016 That Led to the Transformation?

1. Students rebelled against a PowerPoint–dominant, paternalistic, rigid academic medical educational system and demanded more relevant coursework in disparities, cultural competence, and patient skills.

2. The AMERICAN ASSOCIATION OF MEDICAL COLLEGES created a pilot of ten schools that chose students based on self-awareness and empathy. In each of these schools, the percentage of diverse accepted candidates increased exponentially. At the same time, the majority of deans of American medical colleges stopped sending their data to *US News and World Report* to support a "looking to the past" ranking system. At the same time, an independent group developed a "top medical schools of the future" based on parameters that best reflected the need of the present and future.

3. Appointments, promotions, and tenure committees around innovation became the norm such that an individual could advance in an academic institution as a professor of entrepreneurship and innovation based on inventions, patents, commercialization, and creative and meaningful writings.

CHAPTER 15

Of Google, Goggles, and Foggles

*The level of technology used in healthcare today will seem like the dark ages in a few short years. We have to be ready for and embrace that technologic revolution. It needs to start as a blank page. **Michael Dell*** said it back in the 2000s, that as you start your journey, "the first thing you should do is throw away that store-bought map and begin to draw your own." It is great advice for us today as we think about how technology can fundamentally transform how we do things in healthcare, but we have to be creative, bold, **and** accepting of new norms. We talk about GOOGLE glasses and goggles, but none of that technology matters without real vision.*

Whisk, I'm beginning to like this form of travel. Back in the hotel and back in my room. Time is irrelevant, it seems, in this vapor-induced journey, but if perceptions matter, a lot has happened since I woke up this morning. Competence-based testing, simulation, training physicians of the future. All clear and logical and all in just a few hours. On the TV, you guessed it, **Duck Dynasty.**[†] While I don't expect wizard-level wisdom from the **Robertsons**, just as I was about to change the channel, half listening, I heard them say something that, believe it or not, carries a lot of wisdom in our quest for disruption of healthcare.

---

*Michael Dell: the founder and CEO of DELL, INC., who also said, "You don't have to be a genius or a visionary or even a college graduate to be successful. You just need a framework and a dream."

[†] *Duck Dynasty*: an American realty television series on A&E from 2012 to the present. It follows the Robertson family who became wealthy from products for duck hunters, primarily a duck call entitled Duck Commander. It's a wonderful country!

> When you don't know what you're doing, it's best to do it quickly.

Well said, Willie, now there's some wisdom! And while I'm still not ready to binge-watch five seasons of duck hunting escapades, Willie could have been describing my life at the moment. Here we are trying to transform healthcare in a few days, albeit with some real major league guides: a wizard, deans from another decade, and some surreal beings to be named later (no need to guess, they're coming soon).

I headed down to the conference and found the only seat available, this time with the information technology folks. I braced myself and got ready for an enticing discussion about the next hackathon or drone technology.

Actually, the geek squad and the chief medical officer were getting into a pretty good discussion.

Maybe it was part of a dream during a power nap between sessions or simply extended déjà vu from the proceedings of the second day, but the technology equation was suddenly becoming a lot clearer. This morning we had talked about the doctors and other providers. This conversation was all about *patients,* or as much as physicians hated to call them this, our consumers.

And our consumers were already telling us they were "as mad as hell and not going to take it anymore," to quote **Network,** a movie about disruptive change in broadcast journalism in the 1970s.

Shortly before being abducted/invited to this conference, I reviewed surveys in 2015 of patients under age forty and what their expectations were for the immediate consumer-centric technologic changes in healthcare that would better align their health experience with what they had become accustomed to in the rest of their lives. Not surprisingly, they were expecting major changes in how we did business:

- 71 percent expected doctor's offices to have online scheduling with comparative prices by the end of 2016.
- 65 percent expected to have social networking opportunities to discuss health-related topics and *compare* providers, sort of a healthcare equivalent of the very popular student site "rate my professors."

- 92 percent expect to have two-way electronic communication with their providers.

- 83 percent expect to be able to access their health information online with the same ease of access that they have for their bank accounts and travel information.

- 78 percent expect to have total access to family members' inpatient charts and have the ability to virtually or in person participate in rounds.

So what did we do with this incredible shift in consumer/patient expectations. For most of us within the system, not much. There were some people listening, however. It just wasn't centered in our great academic medical centers and community health systems. We were too busy building new inpatient beds (while going to conferences where it was clear we would need fewer inpatient beds) and building hospitals across the street from our competitors in a parochial arms race that (like most arms races) could only result in mutual destruction.

Those pesky entrepreneurs, however, were busy getting ready for a much different future and, once again, counted on those of us responsible for the provision of healthcare to hide our head in the sand while they created companies to satisfy the demand, attract venture capital, and, in some cases, begin the next initial public offering (IPO).

What did we do? Many of us stood on the sidelines until it became obvious that we needed to "buy" the technology because patients' expectations could now be realized. So ZocDoc, TelaDoc, American Well, InTouch Health, NanT Health, EPIC, Athena, and hundreds of other companies took advantage of our inability and unwillingness to acknowledge the new consumer and did it for us—much to their profit.

But the conversation at this breakfast table was decidedly different than the pre-conference "head in the sand" mentality. Realistically, it may have been because instead of having a siloed discussion among geek squad members deciding how technology could help us get closer to a common goal, the vapor mentality allowed for a continuous forum for technological enablers, both from the provider and the information technology space.

Technology was an organic part of the conversation, not an end in and of itself. It was neither the Hail Mary pass at the end of a long, drawn argument nor the oft-perceived impediment to clinical progress. The conversation was, in part, guided by the thoughts from the second day, where we started by acknowledging that healthcare technology will be so fundamentally different in a few years that we, like Michael Dell, would need to throw away that store-bought map and begin by drawing our own map. We would be technological pioneers, borrowing from other industries while also developing our own simple and meaningful technological solutions to common problems.

And, once again, instead of blaming each other, there was a lot of looking in the mirror.

"Look, the gig is up. Consumers will want and will see care in the palm of their hand. They are way ahead of physicians in the desire and willingness to use technology. This better be a wake-up call for us," the chief medical officer continued. "We need a new kind of system that allows us to honor the past and maintain the current record. A system that is one global bucket, reliably holding active, resolved, monitored, and reported information in an intelligent manner that allows us to leverage our collective knowledge for a patient."

The CEO of the Electronic Medical Record (EMR) company—who, pre-vapor, would have been arguing against open-source coding—added, "The inability to have the patient's information owned, managed, and shared intelligently is a barrier that we as vendors need to reimagine in a way that also considers the legal implications of practitioners having potentially unlimited access to vast patient records."

The primary care physician added, "Look, the EMR situation in 2016 is ridiculous, fragmented, and expensive, but it's not all your fault. For a long time, we as clinicians fought any change and refused to be more agile in understanding the larger changes in healthcare outside of the scope of our practice. So we can blame badly implemented and executed Information Systems and Technology (IS&T) plans and software that doesn't work and doesn't communicate across systems, but it was partly because we sat on the sidelines during development."

Now this was getting good.

The EMR CEO, "In an ideal future, we would work together to develop an open system with the goal of true integration. Information would be shared in a way that encourages participation of hospitals, providers, and payors in the aim of improving care and providing transparency."

The insurer walked over to our table, "Only the federal government could mandate a system that would allow for the leverage needed to demand a one-payer, one-system, interoperable solution, but who wants that?!"

"Certainly not the insurers," the neurosurgeon quipped. In this post-vapor environment, that was taken more as a fact than a criticism.

A former federal chief technology officer opined, "Once you open up the floodgates of new technology, patient choice, and democratization and create a situation whereby more of the patients' health and cost for that care are under their control, then the sky is the limit. That is exactly what happened when we went from retirement defined benefit plans to defined contribution 401(k)-type plans. It started a whole new industry of financial advisors who could 'guide' consumers, not tell them what to do. The new healthcare will create digital health advisors who will advise the patient as to how and where to get the best cost/quality ratio based on all available data."

The CEO of a pharmacy conglomerate jumped in, "You are absolutely right, and we are ready to jump into that space. Patients already trust their pharmacist to give them good advice regarding options and cost. The ideal situation would be for us to team up with providers to be that 'certified health planner.' We can be the change agent who will bring about the service features on data and operations that will allow us to bring that UBER-like experience to healthcare."

The patient advocate had been listening in the background. "Look, it's pretty simple—other industries have done it. We need an integrated system that can communicate across patient 'touch points' and allow for an intelligent, living, smart health timeline. Even AMAZON has that for my shopping history. They know every *Star Trek* movie I have bought or **Adele*** CD I own, and they make suggestions. By the way, usually they're right. Why can't my healthcare record do the same thing—include past and present health problems and intelligently link to pertinent follow-up and concrete plans and suggestions specific to me while also tailoring the information so that it is specific to the provider?"

That same contributing author of this book who jumped at us in Chapter 5 once again excitedly launched out of his seat at a low point in the conversation and proclaimed, "What if we all just agree that it is indeed not an electronic medical record owned by the physician but an electronic health record owned by the patient who 'allows' selected physicians to partner with her on her healthcare needs? The provider then is a contributor, not the author, of that record."

The IS&T guru agreed. "Could we challenge ourselves to create an open-source national Electronic Population Health Record that will do those very things that we have always reasonably wanted for ourselves and our patients? Could we ask our mega-EHR-vendors to partner with us in this process, manage parts of this records' development, bring external insights, ensure regulatory compliance, and co-exist with app developers via mass adoption and service and solution selling?"

Admittedly, this fundamentally disruptive point-of-view, absent the collaborative effects of the vapor, would have been scoffed at by vendor and practitioner alike.

But not that day.

That day, it was like a veil was lifted and liberating questions like "how about?" and "what if?" were leading every sentence.

The former chief technology officer of the United States eased into the conversation matter-of-factly by infusing his vision into the proposed solution like we were already building it, right there. Why not, right?

He spoke of the benefits of such a collaborative system, not just to the U.S. population, but to the development of long-term wellness all over the world and the overall productivity of a highly unoptimized

---

* Legendary English singer and songwriter.

system. "We already have the standards, but we have had to approach it with government regulation forcing providers to comply, payers to relent, and patients to wait it out as a status quo solution developed over a long period of time. We don't have to do this if we all agree to put the patient first while building responsible and viable economic models for each of us to thrive."

"Yes, and those models exist in pockets all over the world, in healthcare and outside of it," said a leader of the WORLD HEALTH ORGANIZATION.

The tempo of the conversation really started to accelerate when the CEO of a leading EHR system spoke as a patient and said she owed it to her family and her family's future health to help develop such a visionary system and invited other EHR vendors to join her in this process.

Inspiration flowed out of every corner of the room; from CIOs and CEOs to the banker and lawyer, we realized the obvious—that we are all patients and we can make a technology-enhanced healthcare system the way we want it, both as administrators and stewards of the system and as the recipients of these innovative products. We are all patients and providers, we are all inside and outside the system, and the vapor created some sense out of this very real paradox.

For the first time, many of us recognized the dilemma. The very system we were defending, whatever our role in it, was frustrating as hell when we had to be on the other side of it. With the joint effort of those in the room and others we gathered along our journey, the seeds that were sown during that event iteratively grew into a healthy tree of well-managed lives that, in the last ten years, has led to meaningful insights and breakthroughs in healthcare in the United States and the world over.

From seamless universal systems that enable a patient to register for an appointment with any provider in their region or a specialist anywhere in the nation, to artificial intelligence–enabled (augmented intelligence) systems that share patient data securely and analyze it in real time, in stasis, and longitudinally to decipher patterns and change unhealthy behavior—the future was right in front of our eyes, all the time. We just had to acknowledge the un-mystery to realize it.

For providers, we had true decision support for the first time, the equivalent of computerized systems on airplanes. No, we didn't turn into automatons and all the fears of "cookbook medicine" as naysayers used to call it never materialized, but when a neurosurgeon now walks into an ICU, he/she is no longer depending on intellect and memorization skills to come up with the right decision. There is a true "engine analyzer" that puts the data together with meaningful options. And while it can be overwritten by the human doctor, it's usually right.

It took a while, by the way, to get physicians, especially older physicians to "trust the instruments" as pilots would say. When a pilot is learning how to fly through the clouds, they train with "foggles" over their eyes, glasses that are blacked out except for the bottom so that all you can see is the instruments; the pilot can't see outside. It is very disorienting. The pilot's mind often plays tricks, for example, making him or her believe the plane is going down when it is climbing. But the foggles help them concentrate on and trust the instruments. Many pilot errors happen because they forget that simple fact.

As we developed these decision support systems from 2016 to 2020, we needed to teach physicians, nurses, and other healthcare providers to trust the decision support mechanisms. As you might expect, it took many "virtual foggle sessions" to have those same autonomous, competitive, hierarchical docs "trust the artificial intelligence."

And for all you skeptics out there, rolling your eyes at this optimistic view of the future, there was much *you* contributed after *you* saw some of the early effects of the vision being realized.

Once we moved from electronic *medical* records owned by providers and insurers and maintained by software vendors and moved to electronic *health* records owned by the patient and stored in the cloud, everything changed. Vendors needed to create apps that worked across all records and really provided value either in increased health information to the patient or decision support for the provider. It also shifted power in the doctor–patient relationship from the doctor to the patient. Now if a patient wants to see a different doctor, she doesn't have to go to her previous doctor's office and *hope* that they transfer the records. She owns her record and can just change the password and give that to her new doctor.

That new patient-power shift and movement from legacy systems to a universal health record created an explosion of creativity and entrepreneurism, not seen since APPLE opened the app store on the first iPhone. We revolutionized traditional tele-medicine into a science by adding sensory data and unconventional mashups such as weather stats and pollen counts to better inform the provider about the state of the patient and contributing environmental factors.

Large Internet service providers (ISPs) and cellular network providers then offered their networks and associated intelligence to broaden the reach of tele-medicine to large swaths of the rural United States while also seamlessly connecting urban areas to local tele-medicine hubs to provide prescient, continuous (nonepisodic), and responsive care—all while delivering tremendous value and goodwill to their subscribers. We developed artificial intelligence and cognitive data-processing and decision-making engines that now allow clinicians to focus on the human element and spend time exercising emotional intelligence instead of just engaging in a routine or template assessment. So we now detect early symptoms more accurately and advise patients on their health and wellness more effectively.

New crowd-sourced entrepreneurial models for healthcare data analysis were developed and made available to the world for validation and use via open-source platforms and market places. We developed consumer-driven healthcare front-ends that enabled patients to make quick decisions on their healthcare while enabling them to access the care they needed at any time. More recently, with just three little words spoken into their embedded INTEL voice chips (I Love Me), you can unleash the power of a comforting AMAZON-Alexa-driven, GOOGLE-Organic-Search-enabled, IBM-Watson-analyzed, APPLE-iOS-delivered conduit.* All this at your fingertips to enhance health through low-threshold, always-on, continuous engagement. A long way from the APPLE Watch that detected your steps or **Toby Cosgrove**'s vision of app-mediated EKGs.

---

* Pop-tech life enhancements of 2026.

I could stop this narrative here, but I would then not do justice to the voice of the researcher and educator. The researcher, in true collaborative fashion, provided the backbone for the validation of all our hypotheses and kept us from chasing rainbows by asking us *why* at least five times every time we thought we had found a problem that needed solving. The tele-medicine revolution of 2018 provides a great and instructive example. Tele-health moved from a technology with an attitude to a vehicle that supported the philosophy of getting patients the care they need as close to home as possible. Thus, virtual triage actually potentiated the patients who needed to be seen physically in an emergency room to get the care they needed because the same virtual triage that advised them to go to the ER had already called the ambulance. The ERs were significantly less crowded because deductibles were increased tenfold if a patient did not take advantage of the virtual triage options open to them.

So now a hospital emergency waiting room was filled with true emergencies. The rest had already been virtually sent to urgent care centers, been taken care of remotely, been given an appointment in the morning with their physician, or some combination of the above. It was the health system researchers who sorted out what worked and what did not. It was a great example of the nexus of health systems researchers, with a consumer technology embraced by providers that has now evolved into a true disruption by increasing options and decreasing costs for unscheduled care.

The educators chronicled our achievements and informed the next generation of healthcare innovators and technologists by building our successes and failures into their technology-enhanced, hyper-interactive, immersive, iterative, simulation-driven, and gamified curricula.

As if they could read my mind, one of the "geeks" concluded, "Wow, it sounds like a way brighter future in healthcare technology, I'll need some 2026 SHADES (super hi-def analytic decision engine systems), GOOGLE's next generation goggles turned into organic contact lenses!"

Even the vapor could not prevent the eye-rolling and the references to the fact that not many coders had a future in comedy!

Changes 2016–2026

What's Changed the Most in Technology and Electronic Health Records in 2026?

1. Everyone owns a "must have" multipurpose, elegant, easy-to-use, personal, mobile device with built-in smart health advisor. It is powered by an intelligent agent honed by crowd-sourced literature and source-agnostic-curated information. The electronic health record (owned by the patient) is one of many health information sources for patients. Health service consumers are not waiting to get sick before scrambling to search, research, and schedule appointments with the right caregiver or, for that matter, rush to an emergency center. Instead, they use it as their go-to mobile personal advisor that is built into their smart device. Using this Personal Health Advisor is as easy as saying, "Hello Dr. Zen, I have an unusual reddish rash, what do you advise?" The advisor presents a probable reason and recommends physicians, ranked by community-reported feedback and user's past medical interactions, to reach out and includes a video chat icon to initiate an on-demand tele-health visit.

2. Wearables are omnipresent, and they are integrated into apparel, footwear, and user devices that are connected to smart medical devices that are continuously monitoring fitness and health conditions through wake and sleep states. These devices only intervene when necessary through nudge apps infused with machine-learning, artificial-intelligent agents to keep people healthy and reduce hospital admissions and readmissions. Mega-health facility construction is no longer a norm. Healthcare is a ubiquitous presence on your mobile device, television, and "healthmart" around the corner from where you live.

3. Physicians have multiple personas—physical, avatar, and remote—that are manifested based on consumer health needs. Some of the key criteria for physicians' ranking are their stewardship of personal health and genomics information of patients and their ability to seamlessly interact with their augmented intelligence counterparts.

What Happened in 2016 That Led to the Transformation?

1. Because more than 25 percent of the world population
   and 65 percent of the U.S. population owned smartphones, by
   the end of 2016, and because they were used for all aspects of
   people's lives, a groundswell of demand erupted for coordinated
   virtual health information and care. Any health providers not
   participating in the virtual and tele-health space were left out
   (much like banks that were slow to the consumer and ATM
   movement). Consumerism finally disrupted healthcare as it
   did retail two decades ago.

2. Wearable technology and cognitive sciences matured to be
   useful and affordable and garnered mass appeal, providing a
   perfect recipe for disruptive experimentation and application.
   The wearable craze became the "iPod" of the twenty-first century
   and created unstoppable momentum by the end of 2016. APPLE
   (healthkit, researchkit, and homekit), FITBIT, IBM (Watson),
   GOOGLE (Deep Learning), AMAZON (Echo), and NUANCE
   (Dragon) all became drivers of revenue of the ongoing healthcare technology craze.

3. Health cybersecurity has become the #1 concern of citizens as
   hackers took advantage of the huge datasets available through
   everything from Medicare reporting to APPLE Watch and FITBIT
   information. Some of the fastest rising IPOs were health hacking
   antidote and cybersecurity technology firms.

CHAPTER 16

Of Holiday Shopping and Healthcare

The Great Lie of Patient-Centered Care

Riddle me this: Why can I be sitting in my home the day after Thanksgiving watching **Game of Thrones** *in my pajamas and do ALL of my holiday shopping online, but if I have a stomach ache or a health problem, I can't quickly access a physician or nurse? Even the pharmacy chains have figured it out, it's all about REAL patient service on the same smart device. And my aha moment, post-vapor and blackout, is that a good deal of it is our fault. Yes, us, the patients and consumers. Because we complain about everything in every other aspect of our life, but for fifty years we have tolerated and even promoted lousy service from the healthcare and hospital industry. There was a great series called* **Through the Patient's Eyes** *that recorded the patient's view of what happens in the hospital. We should play that for every physician and hospital CEO to see if that is how they would like to spend their time in the hospital. You as an industry have abandoned all of us during the consumer revolution. How come you can do really cool things in every area of your life: holiday shopping on your iPhone or Android, arrange travel through a variety of e-apps, but you still have to access the healthcare system like you did in the 1990s?*

After day two, I was back in my room and I fell right to sleep. But it didn't last long, my mind was swirling. It's 3 a.m. and I can't sleep. I'm tossing and turning, and every time I fall asleep there's another nightmare about the future. And unlike other sleepless nights, this one is not about the dropping value of my home, my spouse's spending habits, or the aftermath of my neglect to get the dog neutered. In my nightmare, I'm pummeled by a never-ending panoply of initials that make no sense—ACOs, PCMHs, CHIMPs*—not to mention that carpal tunnel syndrome I suffered in my dream from paging through the Affordable Care Act (again), the meaningful use criteria, and the accountable care guidelines. The future seems bleak, empty, and full of stupid regulations and stupider acronyms.

I'm actually considering a sleeping pill, but I know that won't help real estate values, my credit card bills, or my dog's reproductive status.

Fortunately, I remembered that I am at this bizarre conference and I start to head downstairs, sleepwalking-like. (In case you were wondering, I fell asleep in my PHILADELPHIA EAGLES Zubaz pajamas, barely acceptable for sleepwalking in the hotel). Remember this hotel has **Duck Dynasty** on almost nonstop, so formal sleepwalking gear is not required.

I'm in the conference room. The tables. The whiteboards. By myself.

In my dream?

I am almost blinded by the headlights. Up to the podium walks a guy that reminded me of **Dr. Emmett Brown**† from *Back to the Future*—that

---

* ACO: accountable care organization; groups of doctors, hospitals, and other healthcare providers who come together voluntarily to give coordinated, high-quality care to their Medicare patients; helped organizations get through the "twilight zone of healthcare"; virtually abandoned experiment by 2019.

PCMH: patient-centered medical home; care delivery model whereby patient treatment is coordinated through primary care physicians to ensure patients receive the necessary care when and where they need it, in a manner they can understand; basically a name for care that should have been coordinated through a family physician long ago.

CHIMPS: changes in mandatory programs; nothing to do with the cute human-like animals, rather, everything to do with legislators not wanting to take on Medicare and Social Security.

† Doc Brown: In the movie *Back to the Future*, a science fiction adventure comedy. Christopher Lloyd played Doc Brown, the fictional inventor of the first time machine, which he builds out of a Delorean sports car. The real Doc Brown did not visit the future of healthcare.

1980s movie where a self-described crazy astrophysicist befriends a high school student and has him choose and help determine two alternate futures. All you had to do was get in a Delorean, a car that only started half the time for normal people, get to 88 miles per hour in a shopping mall parking lot. Yes, you *could* get away with that kind of stuff in the 1980s!

As I was trying to remember other bad movies of the 1980s (think **Jaws 3, Cannonball Run, Galaxina, Mac and Me,** and **The Happy Hooker Goes Hollywood**), the lights went on and my conference colleagues were all here. Not sure if I had fallen back asleep or the whole thing was a daydream and I had never gone back to my room.

Looking down on my EAGLES Zubaz helped me resolve that mystery.

And there he was. Not Doc Brown, but an astrophysicist ready to take us—where?

"Great Scott!" the astrophysicist began. "A wizard asked me to come here and help you get to an optimistic future in healthcare. I've scouted it out for you. There are two very different healthcare futures: an amazing patient-centric future in which technology and humanism, patients and providers have created an ideal partnership. And a pessimistic, depressing "nothing has changed" future in which policymakers are still bickering, physicians are still autonomous and competitive, and patients still cannot do half the cool things in healthcare that they can do in the rest of their lives. According to my calculations, *this* room is the key."

"Wait, haven't we seen this movie before? Literally!" exclaimed the pharma executive.

"Yes you have, but for years, you have put billboards up extolling your 'patient-centric healthcare'—and it was all a ruse. So it's time to decide: Which future do you want?" the astrophysicist exclaimed boldly.

"I don't think that's fair," the primary care doc jumped up. "We care about patients. That's why we went into healthcare."

Now the patient advocate got into the fray. "I'm sure you do care. But why should a patient with cancer agonizing in their home on a snowy day have to travel to an office and sit in a waiting room? Why should a mother with a crying baby who can't make an early appointment with her primary care provider have to go to the emergency room and get a bill that will bankrupt the family budget?"

"She's right," said the chief medical officer. "My hospital put bill-boards all around the city because we are now doing 'virtual rounds.' We recognized that it is absurd that if you have a parent in a cancer center and you are not in that city, you still have to call your mom or dad and ask *them* what the doctor said. So we started virtual rounds, where loved ones can participate in a two-way discussion during rounds. It was heralded in *Forbes* magazine as a great "innovation." I was proud of myself for about two minutes. And then I said, damn we could have done this five years ago with Facetime, ten years ago with SKYPE, or twenty years ago on the telephone. But we didn't."

"Exactly," said the astrophysicist. "Great Guns, you are at a nexus point in the time–space continuum. Either you get it right now or the whole American healthcare establishment will go the way of BLOCK-BUSTER and KODAK and be taken over by large multinational noncreative corporations. Of course, that's the worst-case scenario."

Well, it was like opening up a floodgate.

The patient advocates who were also at **President Obama**'s first conference (the one in 2008 sans vapor, blackouts, or self-reflection) turned out to be the most angry of us all.

"The healthcare system is a maze," they said. "It's impossible to get a health insurance issue resolved. It's impossible to get a bill you believe. I had a bill sent to a collection agency because the insurance company put it down as a car accident when I was nowhere near a car. They were trying to get the automobile insurance to pay it. Then I call and they say, sorry, but it will take ten days to fix it. So I call back ten days later, and no one has done anything, so it takes another ten days."

"It's physically intimidating. I have to drive, take a bus, or get trans-port, to a facility where I get lost, where I wait, where I'm treated like it's a factory. When I finally do get to see the doctor, it's made clear to me that I should feel lucky to see him. He is overwhelmed today. Too many patients were scheduled. The office is changing over to a new electronic health record system and everything's delayed. And, you know, he is one of the best specialists in the country."

The temperature in the room was rising. "It is bizarre, especially at academic medical centers, that you are constantly reminded how lucky you are to be *there* seeing *that* physician—for something I am *paying* for. I saw **Andrea Bocelli** last weekend and they thanked *me* for coming. They didn't tell me how lucky I was to be seeing one of the greatest tenors in the world!"

Pile on time.

"Repeatedly I'm ordered to get a test, or x-ray, or even a procedure that appears to be defensive medicine. Do they know it takes four days to get a simple procedure? A trip to the blood-draw facility. A trip to the radiology facility. A pre-op visit. A day at the ambulatory surgery center, most of it spent waiting. A post-op visit. That's a week of sick time, or it's a week without pay! Why can't they coordinate the care and bring it to me?" Another patient heard from.

"Why can't I just call or email a doctor without having to go through a ridiculous set of options, often to end up with an answering machine, service, or someone who can't answer my question?" The complaints were reaching a fever pitch.

And then one patient said he noticed if he used a tele-health app, he could talk to an emergency room physician in seconds, faster than if he went to an emergency room. Faster than he could make an appointment with a primary care physician. And for many ailments, most of the visit could be conducted in that one conversation—almost instantly.

Why wait days for an appointment just to be told you need a blood test? Why not have that consultation on the phone and then use another phone call to talk about the blood test results?

Another patient tried the nurse practitioner at the local pharmacy. It worked. She got evaluated and treated faster than a drive to her doctor's office.

"Great Bones. It sounds like the bad future is already here. We need to find out what you need to do to get to a consumer-friendly, primary care–driven, technology-savvy, alternate scenario." Zap!

In an instance, we were virtually watching some patient encounters from sometime in the future.

Our guide looked confused. "According to my calculations, this is the future in which you never had this conference."

Sure enough nothing had changed.

In the ultimate mystery shopping experience, we were actually watching a real patient encounter in the bad alternate 2026, where the conference had never happened and nothing had changed.

We were in a busy hospital emergency center. We've all been there, people of all sizes and shapes, creeds and colors, coughing, bleeding, but mostly waiting. And waiting. And waiting. We watched as a child with a rash all over her body who had been waiting with the other children in the ER get seen by the doctor.

After about a four-hour wait, the physician says to the crying child's mother, "Rachel has chicken pox, we will call something in to make her feel more comfortable, and I will have your pediatrician see you in his office tomorrow. Now I have to just hope that everyone else in the waiting room has had chicken pox or been immunized because they are all at risk."

Our astrophysicist guide showed up in a white coat. "With all the technology that exists today, something that could have been diagnosed by sight and tele-health required a patient to drive to the emergency center, spend five hours with a crying child and a few hundred dollars or more, and potentially infect some other children and adults."

Before we could even react, we were whisked away, this time to a large football stadium, Gillette Stadium, in 2016 where the NEW ENGLAND PATRIOTS were playing the PHILADELPHIA EAGLES.

"Why are we here?" asked the small business CEO—a perfectly logical question.

"Because before I take you to the good alternate future where you see the fruits of your labor after the conference, I want you to see how far healthcare has been surpassed by every other aspect of society. Great Scott, even if we didn't have this nifty form of travel, we could have Ubered you to this game after we bought tickets with one click on one of many ticket sites."

Our guide continued, "If you weren't invisible and wanted a beer, you would no longer have to wave your hand, pass cash down to a vendor, and have it spill on everyone before it gets to you. There is an app that allows you to pay for the beer and have it delivered cashlessly. Oh, and by the way, there are six guys with computers up there mapping every play, every down and determining the probabilities based on mathematical modeling of what plays will succeed. Simply put, **Tom Brady** has a better idea of whether or not a screen pass will work than your doctors do of what cancer drug is best or whether a patient should be in hospice or the ICU for end-of-life care or what factor gives a patient the greatest chance of being readmitted for heart failure."

Yes, this was embarrassing. NFL football is more customer centric, is technologically advanced, and has better predictive tools than American healthcare in 2016.

Just as I was pondering the enormity of that discrepancy, our guide said. "Great Scott, it's time for us to go. By the way, the EAGLES win by 10!"

CHAPTER 17

Doc Well and the Optimistic
Future of Healthcare

Fast forward: We were whisked away. This time clearly to the future, or at least to our current time, 2026.

Ladies and Gentlemen, welcome to the *optimistic* alternate future.

We were in some kind of nerve center with nurses and physicians talking to patients on large screens and pharmacists wirelessly prescribing and filling medications.

A young physician stepped up—actually gave me a flashback to the McFly version of **Michael J. Fox** from the 1980s movie or, more accurately, **Doc Hollywood**.

"Welcome to the new healthcare future you helped create," the new doctor began optimistically. "**I'm Doc Well.** In this future, the health system and the payors are aligned, and oddly enough, the answer is not in a shiny new hospital or new ICU; the answer is not in expanding our emergency room or building new operating rooms. The answer is in the last place you would have expected to see it back in the first two decades of the twenty-first century. The answer starts in the patient's home and then extends as a partnership with her patient-centered medical home, with her healthcare coach and extensivist, with her primary care team and their tele-health partners, and their related specialists, and with a new type of creative partnership with the payors who provide decision support to promote 'optimal utilization.' That means in 2016 you did a great job of promoting overutilization and underutilization but never 'doing the right procedure for the right patient at the right time.'

"Let me introduce to you the chief medical officer [CMO] of this place, what used to be called Pleasantville General Hospital but now encompasses a much larger system titled the Pleasantville Community Centers of Well-Being of which the inpatient centers are much smaller and have gone from revenue centers to cost centers for very complex cased and for failed health and wellness initiatives."

"Welcome," started the optimistic CMO. As we were preparing for your visit, my colleagues and I were laughing at the reception last night about how ten years ago we spent the majority of our energy on the inpatient units of our health system and the majority of time with our physicians on credentialing and quality issues (mostly after an error had already occurred) in our inpatient units. As senior managers of the Pleasantville Community Centers of Well-Being, aka Pleasantville General Hospital, we were excited to look back on the most significant changes that occurred once we started to partner with the community, promote health, and recognize that you could, indeed, bend the cost curve by providing better care at a lower cost by concentrating on keeping the patients of Pleasantville healthier.

"We never would have imagined that, as a senior manager of a hospital, we would have been dealing with wireless scales in patients' homes, healthcare coaches, and electronic learning centers. Now that Pleasantville has been deemed one of 'America's Healthiest Hometowns,' I am excited to show you what's changed over the last ten years."

"How did *we* help make this happen?" the insurance executive asked the question that was on all of our minds.

"Once you returned to your hometowns from the famous 'black-out–no blame' conference and each of you went around the country talking about the alternate pessimistic and optimistic futures, we all went to work," Doc Well said with some degree of awe and reverence.

"You guys were the pioneers, the potentiators. Government helped it all hit the fan when joint replacements and some other 'low-hanging fruit' admissions became outpatient procedures and hospitals that had not prepared for disruption were caught flat-footed. For God's sake, back in 2016, there were still some academic medical centers building new inpatient towers, assuming that the 'hub-and-spoke' model where patients would be sent from community hospitals to high-cost academic medical centers would just continue forever.

"Of course, the government helped by creating innovation grants for hospitals that were willing to ask the tough questions and 'dream' about how to get to that future. I still remember the first grant we got back in 2017. We had a get-together and, after a nice dinner (and a few drinks), we asked our senior managers to get out of their 2017 mindset and, with no constraints, imagine a different, optimistic healthcare future by imagining they were here in 2026 and talking about what has changed specifically over the last ten years as it relates to physician alignment, ambulatory operations, medical staff bylaws, information systems, and care coordination between 2017 and this new present. We concentrated on:

- Partnerships with Pleasantville that result in care that is patient-centric, community based, primary care driven, innovative, and integrated that we might not have envisioned in 2017.

- Differential payment rates based on quality initiatives and outcomes that fundamentally and nonincrementally bent the cost curve.

- Relative revenue based on inpatient and outpatient activity as well as new sources of revenue in this community partnership.

- How to best position the system to work jointly with our physicians to accept responsibility for the quality and cost of care for a panel of patients.

- Changes in our medical staff and bylaws as well as physician employment models that we would not have predicted in 2017.

- The expanded role of nonphysician providers and new types of healthcare professionals in this community partnership.

- The role of prevention and wellness programs and 'patient responsibility' in decreasing overall healthcare costs.

- The significant changes that occurred that resulted in better alignment of physician and provider incentives with the goals of the patient, the organization, and the community.

"Not as fancy as a Delorean at 88 miles an hour but, believe it or not, the fact that your group helped to allay some of the pessimism and posit an optimistic disruptive future started a positive feedback cycle that has resulted in our new patient-centric future." Well was on a roll.

"We even got our board on the Back to the Optimistic Healthcare Future train," he said.

The trustees went through some of the greatest changes. They, too, were laughing at the reception last night in preparation for your visit how they oversaw a disconnect between *missions* that were quality- and community engagement–driven but spent most of their time at board meetings listening to reports on inpatient census and self-congratulatory statements that there had been 10 percent fewer hospital-acquired infections."

"By the way," a new, young white coat entered the room. "Hospital-acquired infections are now reportable events. I think the last time we had one was 2023, once patients were allowed to charge the hospitals for lost time, lost wages, etc. Literally, all it took was a service guarantee and penalty. The hospitals that couldn't move to zero defects closed or were merged with the ones that had figured it out."

Doc Well continued, "They recognized that the role of a trustee needed to go through some of the same disruptions that patients, administrators, doctors, nurses, and others were experiencing. They were part of the problem—and part of the solution."

"So we went through the same 'virtual colonoscopy' that our docs and administrators went through, and believe me it was painful." This from a distinguished older gentleman who identified himself as an "old country car dealer." He was actually one of the most successful manned and unmanned drone dealers in the United States (who had started his career as a "Kia dealer" in Florida), but had made most of his money starting a chain of virtual car dealerships that made ordering a car as easy as streaming movies onto your TV. More importantly, he was chair of the board at Pleasantville General.

"We took our role as a board leading an industry through transformation seriously. We asked and answered some of these tough questions," he continued.

- How can we continue to pretend that job #1 was quality when that was a small percentage of the CEO and other senior manager's incentives?

"I used to say, if you want to know what your hospital will look like ten years from now, don't look at the mission and vision. Look at the CEO's incentives. If the incentives are about census, (EBITA) earnings before interest, taxes, and amortization, and bond rating and your mission is around top quality, reducing health disparities, and community engagement, then guess what? You will have a hospital with a high hospital census, great bond rating, and increasing EBITA. Health equality, zero defects, community hiring, diversity, and involvement—not so much!"

- How did we engage the community to understand the necessary changes in their behavior and attitude toward the hospital system?
- How did we measure our progress in promoting best outcomes out in the community when home and ambulatory sites have taken an increased role?

As I was contemplating how all these changes could have occurred in my time frame without supernatural involvement, the neurosurgeon from our group picked up a magazine that was laying on the desk: *US News and Interplanetary Report (USNIR)*: "Best Hospitals and Medical Schools—2026."

Changes 2016–2026

What's Changed the Most in Patient-Centered Care and the Role of Hospitals, Senior Leaders, and Trustees in Healthcare?

1. Health systems are no longer "anchored" by expensive, high-fixed-cost hospitals but are now community centers of well-being and portals of care.

2. The health system is led by a senior administrator in tandem with a "CEO of patients." This CEO of patients stands on equal footing with the traditional chief executive officer, usually comes from a customer service (non-healthcare) background, and is responsible for all patient experience aspects of the system.

3. Trustees for most non-profit health systems include patient advocates and traditional community business leaders, but almost half are recruited nationally for their expertise in quality,

information technology, health disparities, innovation, and other areas usually not represented in the governance of non-profit health systems.

What Happened in 2016 That Led to the Transformation?

1. High deductible plans and increased movement to ambulatory (non-inpatient-stay) procedures forced hospitals that had "doubled down" on inpatient beds to be acquired or repurposed. Subsequent sophisticated connection of personal health management and financial risk completed the transformation.

2. Metahealthcritic.com, a compendium of all available data regarding quality, service, food, cost, friendliness of staff, errors, cleanliness, and waiting times for doctors and hospitals, became the must-have app of 2016. As data became more available, patients increasingly made decisions for care based on this objective data.

3. The large health system consolidations that survived shared these qualities: high quality–low cost in the market, their academic medical center "flagships" went from revenue centers to cost centers, patient-centered care meant the abolition of traditional department structures, and a full commitment to service lines and centers of excellence and capital investments increasingly came through creative partnerships with private equity, industry, and venture philanthropy.

CHAPTER 18

Hospital and University Rankings

Other Planets Weigh In

"This should be interesting" he mused. "My guess is that *US News and World Report* rankings are one thing that *hasn't* changed."

He couldn't have been more wrong. Actually, the opening page said it all:

Celebrating the Tenth Anniversary of the New "Best Of"
Parameters

It is amazing how far we have come toward "accurately" reflecting the academic and healthcare organizations of excellence based on the issues that really matter to students and patients as opposed to an idealized picture of the past that rewarded those academic and healthcare entities for doing "more of the same" while resisting any disruptive changes toward the future.

Even our magazine's title has changed, recognizing the discovery within the last five years of other inhabited planets with their own imperfect academic and healthcare institutions.

"Guess I should have noticed the title change," the neurosurgeon exclaimed.

"It must have started with those brave deans in 2018 who refused to send their database to the old *US News and World Report* database, that old system that we heard about from **Dean Wurmer**," our own 2016 dean interjected.

"Apparently one of those planets actually abducted a medical student and brought her back with the knowledge she should have learned in medical school," exclaimed one of the authors of this book in a shameless reference to a previous book written by us.*

The opening page continued:

Here are the five academic and five healthcare parameters leading to "best of" status that have changed the most in the last ten years:

Medical Colleges

Personal and professional outcomes at one year, three years, and five years: Since universities used to charge an obscene tuition with no real follow-up or incentive for individual student success (which is why we should not have universities in the first place), our rankings are now heavily weighted toward a survey mechanism measuring an individual's professional and personal happiness at varying intervals after graduation.

Collaborative quotient: While ten years ago there was almost no incentive for universities or medical centers to work with each other, we have now recognized that the arms race between academic entities within shouting distance of each other just served to raise costs and did little to improve outcomes. We now give "extra points" to those academic entities that "get over themselves" and work well with others.

Entrepreneurial quotient: Ten years ago the "e" word was discouraged as a measure of academic or hospital success. Today, we reward those institutions that have invented and envisioned new ways of doing things that bring in alternative sources of revenue to fund growth and create business opportunities.

Coolness factor: This one is simple. We recognized, here at *USNIR*, that we often had a group of sixty-somethings ranking schools that would be teaching twenty-somethings. We now have a separate panel of recently graduated students that assesses how technology is utilized to "make learning fun."

Disruptive quotient: Extra credit is given to those academic entities that invested in and created ideas that may fundamentally transform an area of interest. This quotient is not dependent on

---

* *The Phantom Stethoscope: A Field Manual for Finding an Optimistic Future in Medicine,* Hillsboro Press, 1999.

success or failure, just an attempt to be disruptive that has others thinking differently.

Hospitals and Health Systems:

The "BUB" quotient: This is a formula that did not even exist in our rankings for 2016, but it is the "believable understandable bill" quotient. It reflects an understanding that the absurd, non-readable bills that patients have previously been subjected to reflect a larger disregard for your customer base.

The "before I go to sleep, does the Doc know what he's doing" quotient: This is another new factor that replaces the "making never events never happen" quotient that we instituted in 2017. Simply put, hospitals are rewarded who objectively validate their surgeons as "competence certified" in each of the procedures they perform.

The "follow the yellow brick road" factor: This is another one of our new "being patient centric is not just marketing" parameters. We hire random people of average intelligence and good eyesight to navigate the halls of your hospital and "find" various important areas, such as nursing stations, ERs, ORs, etc., based on available wayfinding. There is also a diversity component (we hire surveyors who speak the top three languages spoken in your service area). Extra points are given for helpful "guides" (human or otherwise) that can speak several languages.

The "say what you mean and mean what you say" quality parameter: This research for "best of" has been a boon for graduates of marketing and communications programs. We hire those types of individuals to read all the hospital's billboards, news ads, social marketing, and Web claims and investigate them for any semblance of truth and/or relevance. Any health systems that grade "below zero" for these elements are transferred to the "quality fraud" section of the magazine.

The "through the patient's eyes" factor: Thanks to new technology that allows us to film hospital interactions directly from the patient's vantage point (GOOGLE glasses were an early iteration), literally through the patient's eyes, we now take ten random samplings from each hospital and have other hospital CEOs watch the interactions and grade each from one to ten based on the "would I want to be treated that way?" scale.

"It's hard to believe that, barely ten years ago, we were rating universities and health systems based on decades-old parameters that had little to do with the actual patient or student experience," **Doc Well** of 2016 explained. "Progress is grand. Now if I could only get my TESLA hovercraft fixed!" A quick glance at his board chair, the "old country car dealer."

CHAPTER 19

Betting the Pharma on a New Healthcare Solution

[So sayeth the CEO of one of the world's largest pharma companies:] I need to move from selling medical devices and specialty pharmaceuticals to being part of the solution team. If my products, data, and expertise can help our customers (who are both patients and providers) have better care at a lower cost, that will be good for healthcare and good for business. Between us and the large pharmacy providers, such as my friend over in the third row who oversees the largest pharmacy chain in America, we know more about the patient than her provider or hospital does. By the way, truth be told, I didn't need the vapor and blackout to convince me. I was already realizing that if I am just selling commodities, someone will undercut me. I need new kinds of partnerships with health systems, universities, and patients in order to be a driver of the optimistic future.

A physician in her thirties spoke in a very serious tone. "Guides! Thank you." Then, "I am very hopeful you can convince your emissaries from 2016 to move toward this optimistic future. My dad was a doc in your era, and he talked about how tele-health was viewed as a gimmick, how states created barriers to its use, and how *more* care was considered *better* care. It seems medieval to us now. It's not just access to healthcare, it's access to health.

"The real change was when we stopped looking at technologies like tele-health or enterprise internet scheduling as an end in themselves, but rather as a means to embolden patients' relationships with their existing care teams," she continued. "From what I understand from my dad, our visitors from 2016 came away from some kind of secret conference and led the way in educating patients as to how they can start to be aware and engaged in these human–technology relationships."

"As one of your participants said after the conference," Doc Well agreed, looking at us, "in a statement that was quoted heavily in the elections of 2016, 'It's time to bring medicine home. To be truly patient-centric, we need to think about the patient before he or she leaves home, not just when the patient is in the doctor's office or hospital.'

"Creative partnerships were a key—patient/provider, industry/academic, entrepreneur/researcher. Perfect timing . . ." Doc Well was interrupted by another board member who had just entered the room, the CEO of a large multinational pharma company.

He didn't waste any time.

"As it turned out, the future belonged to a partnership of clinicians, entrepreneurs, industry, and patients. Patients who 'plug in,' who engage in self-service, who go online, who join social media and virtual support groups have better health outcomes than patients who don't. Isolation kills. Connectivity is good medicine. Taking ownership is the single greatest step toward health and wellness.

"There developed an interesting and growing role for business in this shift. These new alliances changed how healthcare was delivered. The trick was to match the consumer movement of engaged patients with the developing new platforms for care. It was an exciting time, from 2016 to 2019, a chance for us to work together to make significant advances in health."

He continued, "We realized that if all we were doing was selling Band-Aids for $2.95 or laparoscopic equipment for $2.95 million, then I was doomed to be in the commodity business, and my relevance and profits would continue to erode.

"So, we made a decision to be in the *solutions* business. Our sales force evolved into a *solutions* force that, as systems enlarged, became intimately involved with our 'customer.' We embedded members of our sales team into the culture and organization of these large systems and, after the gainsharing legislation of 2017, in which policymakers recognized that many of the regulations meant to protect consumers were actually making it *more* difficult to move from volume to value, we were able to adjust our pricing and profit strategy in order to have 'skin in the game' along with our provider and system partners. If I truly believe that my device or drug is the most efficient, effective path to wellness and creates the most value, then I was part of the 'team' that made that happen and my success was tied to those results.

"I see in this change a parallel with what you called coming out of your conference 'moving from BLOCKBUSTER to NETFLIX.' Medicine headed for the NETFLIX model. It came home. Schools, malls, convenience stores, homes, and mobile anywhere shaped a model that provided care to consumers when, how, and where they wanted it. This shift could have happened during your time, but I think traditional health systems had been smug and, frankly, hadn't had any competition.

"Now they have lots of competition. That competition is not coming from other health systems, but rather from WALGREENS, WALMART, and serial entrepreneurs who were used to traditional health systems standing by while they worked to disrupt the hospital-centric model. A lot of folks cashed in as the patient-as-consumer movement grew, and the need to offer help to people outside of doctors' offices couldn't be clearer. Some of you got it and prospered, and other health systems kept building inpatient beds and figured they could turn on the light switch when the payment system moved from volume to value, from physician-as-customer to patient as customer. By that time, it was way too late, and they are now highlighted in the 'Good to Gone' history books of 2026.

"Even back in your time, while we erroneously thought of medicine as based in hospitals, in fact, 84 percent of America's health costs were incurred fighting chronic illnesses, the kind that can diminish quality of life for years. This was true for the entire population, not just the elderly or under-resourced. While hospitals and clinics remained the place for acute, critical intervention, living with these illnesses happened outside of doctors' offices.

"For example, a Type 1 diabetic patient makes more than two hundred health decisions every day around eating, drinking, exercising, driving, sleeping, and even engaging in sexual relations.

"The traditional healthcare industry was the last to recognize that was where the 'action' was. They missed the whole 'upstream medicine' thing. Population health and financial management demanded a broader, more holistic focus on the member. Integrated, multidisciplinary care teams replaced the provider-centric model. Consumers began to own their medical record and had much more control over their health and treatment. Patient satisfaction became *the* critical metric. Systems married consumer with clinical, claims, and wearable data to create actionable master records that helped providers manage patients throughout the ecosystem. Members of the population then became segmented to narrow characteristics, and systems strived for 'N = 1' precision, where a 'segment' became defined as an individual member.

"These daily decisions about health drove the demand for greater control and self-service in healthcare. The fastest capitalized startup in healthcare in your era was THERANOS, founded by **Elizabeth Holmes**,* which ramped up fast and became controversial even faster. But she argued it was a fundamental right for people to have access to lab and blood testing for themselves. Now the concept of waiting for a physician to *order* a blood test is as antiquated as downloading music physically onto a hard drive.

"The revolution in the relationship among industry, healthcare, and academia started in late 2017, when it became obvious that if the legacy organizations were to survive, they needed a new model, new ways to

---

* Elizabeth Holmes: an American billionaire businesswoman, and the CEO of Theranos, a blood test company founded in 2003. The company hopes to give consumers more power over their own blood tests by making it easier to order tests and obtain results directly.

work together to manage potential conflicts of interest, competitive secrecy, and still speed the revolution of knowledge to advancing health. Some of these models were 'pre-competitive,' where basic research was supported and sped up by collaboration. Some models involved multiuniversity consortia that collected big data but contracted it out as collaborators pursued product development.

"Nationally, business investment attracted to these new delivery platforms became substantial, and there were new winners and losers among industry and academia, not based on past reputation or traditional parameters, but on speed, flexibility, and creative partnerships. BLOOMBERG and a group of consultants looked at the GLOBAL INNOVATION 1000* companies in your era and found that $13.8 billion of their research and development expenditures were in 'digital enablers' for healthcare. That was half the budget of the entire NATIONAL INSTITUTES OF HEALTH of your era, and it grew much faster.

"The universities you are reading about in the 2026 US News and Inter planetary Report (*USNIR*)** 'Top 50' are the ones that figured out that we were going through a nexus of change. They figured out that entrepreneurship and academics were not mutually exclusive. They had been averse to risk and suspicious of profit, sometimes with good reason. But innovation became *the* mission for higher education, and innovation meant flexibility, speed, and the ability to take risk. We needed tenure and promotion criteria to include entrepreneurship and innovation. And we needed structures for faculty to share in return from risk, while providing a clear picture of potential conflicts of interest.

"We recognized the need to ensure our brightest students and young scientists are trained to lead the revolution, not become frustrated by their training. An editorial by **Alan Leshner**, the former CEO of the AMERICAN ASSOCIATION FOR THE ADVANCEMENT OF SCIENCE

---

* Global Innovation 1000: studies begun by PWC that, every year since 2005, investigate the relationship between how much companies spend on research and development and what their overall financial performance is. Every year, the study reinforces the conclusion that there is no statistically significant relationship between the two.

** US News and Interplanetary Report, evaluating universities throughout the known worlds.

hit the nail on the head. He started by observing that in the United States, more than 60 percent of new PhDs in science 'will not have careers in academic research, yet graduate training in science has followed the same basic format for almost one hundred years, heavily focused on producing academic researchers.' He concluded that 'the system is failing to meet the needs of the majority of its students.'"

"He was right!" Doc Well maintained.

"The successful universities recognized the need to partner with industry to develop students with the skills for the emerging health professions, for the workforce of the future," the 2026 pharma CEO and trustee agreed.

"The healthcare industry, even back in 2016, was desperately unable to find skilled professionals who could combine big data and user experience. We needed engineers who understood the predictive analytics of genomics, population health, and user design. And we needed professionals who could help patients make meaning from knowledge. We knew there was a revolution waiting to happen if we could empower patients," he said passionately.

"But your tools at the time to help patients take control of their health were clumsy, relying on exercise trackers when you needed life changers," he continued. "But many universities continued to hang on to the old model, with tenured professors hanging on to the way they did it in their era.

"So, pharma, medical device companies, and others in the healthcare arena found some willing university partners to help them create the workforce of the future. New for profit–non-profit models and unusual partnerships emerged. Pharmaceutical companies, for example, were struggling to offer more than pills, to use their knowledge to guide behavior as well as provide medication. But we didn't have the workforce to take that big step, to enhance health, not just provide the drugs.

"Many universities did not want to enter the 'dark side' of an industry–academic partnership. They missed the boat, or the spaceship as it were. The universities now at the top of the USNIR rankings took on that challenge, to speed up the emerging health professions that take this rush of scientific discovery and translate it into lifestyle and population health.

"The smart universities dismantled their tenure systems and created new blueprints for strategic action, recognizing that they had a dual mission. On the one hand, we needed the next generation of bench laboratory researchers, those who will lead the science of the future. At the same time, we needed scientists who could figure out how to bring those breakthroughs from the laboratory bench, not just to the hospital bedside, but to the home, where people struggle with their illnesses and their health. Those INSTITUTES FOR EMERGING HEALTH PROFESSIONS created new degrees, partly funded by those of us in pharma and other industries that needed those students with training for the future, from forensics to genomics to habit change to 'trusted health advisors.' These creative partnerships, which would have been looked down upon in the early twenty-first century, became the driver for the health science universities of the future."

The dean from our group noted, "I was surprised that some of the universities that were consistently at the top of the 'old rankings' were not there in the USNIR best of list. And others seemed to be 'hyphenated,' indicating creative partnerships, JACK WELCH MANAGEMENT INSTITUTE/THOMAS JEFFERSON UNIVERSITY, JOHNSON AND JOHNSON/BOSTON UNIVERSITY, EPIC/UNIVERSITY OF WISCONSIN, to name a few."

Doc Well summed it up. "Still, what we see as routine today was surprising during your time, a complete transformation of the platforms on which healthcare is delivered. The future of health belonged to patients 'owning' their own health, at home, in their neighborhoods and communities. We needed a generation of bright young scientists to help us make that happen."

The pharma CEO smiled and said, "former APPLE CEO, **John Sculley**, got it right when he posted on TWITTER that 'tele' will be dropped from tele-health just like online was dropped from online banking."

"He hit the nail on the head," Doc Well continued. "Not about TWITTER, that is now an historical footnote, but about the future platforms for healthcare. What we now take for granted was still being debated back in your time. We look at your lack of consumer focus as the medical equivalent of the pre-antibiotic era."

"Great," interrupted the insurance exec from our era. "I always wanted to be equated with the blood-letters of the nineteenth century and the pre-antibiotic era."

"Listening to this guy, I feel like those docs in the SHOWTIME series *The Knick*, where they did surgery with no gloves in their suits and ties," mused the neurosurgeon.

"This guy" from 2026, the pharma exec, continued, "Sorry to say this, but you're not that far off. What is routine to us was 'disruptive' and even 'laughed off' from some of the extinct leaders of your time. Here's a few:

- On-demand health.
- Streaming data between doctors and patients during daily activity.
- Retail medicine in convenient neighborhood locations, including grocery stores and pharmacies.
- Self-service medicine aimed at wellness.
- Patient ownership of doctor's notes, tests, and the hospital electronic health record.
- Tele-health, which now is as common as ATMs.

"Actually there was a great 'back in the 2010s' exposé on ALL-FLIX about banking and healthcare. When online banking and ATMs came into vogue, your grandparents were skeptical. How can the machine access my account? Is it secure? Will they steal my money? In 2016, you laugh at that mentality. This documentary traced the same attitude in the 2010s about retail health and tele-health. States enacting different rules. Questions about payment and security. Sorry to say this, but in ten short years, the debates you folks are having have become head-scratching history."

The physician CEO of a storied academic medical center of our group, probably the most conservative of us when the conference started, made a statement that was every bit as bold as any revolutionary cry, "I can attest that when I get back, we are not going to stand by like BLOCKBUSTER while others disrupt the industry. At my university and health system, our definition of success will move from how many beds are filled in our hospitals to how can I 'stream' our care out to where patients work and live through enabling technologies. This seems like good health and good business!"

CHAPTER 20

Of Alt-Uber and Emerging Health Professions

A nd so that's how bloodless revolutions begin. The Healthcare Revolution of 2016 was officially under way.

Some health systems apparently embraced it; others laughed and continued to build inpatient beds and ignore the consumer revolution.

"Was this an evolution or a revolution?" the health system CEO asked, obviously trying to understand what could possibly get him to view his keystone hospital as anything other than a flagship revenue center.

Doc Well had the clear answer, almost anticipating the question. "In 2018, when joint replacements became an outpatient procedure, those hospitals and health systems that had ignored the transformation and assumed if the world changed they would just react, had to close their doors. Like any transformations—BLOCKBUSTER to NETFLIX, KODAK film to digital cameras—there were enough warning signs, and ignoring them occurred at your own risk and often led to extinction.

"It got down to the fact that patients wanted care when and where they wanted it, and the increased prevalence of high-deductible insurance plans have changed the whole ball game. Patients can now make decisions based on a Match.com type of parameter if they need care or a procedure. There are several "health advisor" apps (similar to TRIP ADVISOR or YELP of your time) that match the out-of-pocket expenses with objective metrics around quality, location, and even ZAGAT-type information such as friendliness of the staff, cleanliness of waiting rooms, etc.*

"The thought of making a decision as to which hospital to go to or what doctor to do your surgery based on no data and a single recommendation is as archaic as physical car dealerships."

A quick glance at his board chair who had made his fortune turning car buying into a consumer sport.

"I believe in your time we hadn't gotten to the TESLA model of ordering all cars online and having them show up, customized to your home," he added, eliciting a wry smile from his chair.

"Most of our post-op checks are virtual now, which has decreased readmissions and increased patient compliance and engagement. We have a virtual triage function, which has gone a long way to reducing preventable emergency department use. That became especially important when many insurers increased deductibles for high-acuity emergency visits to a thousand dollars if the patient did not go through virtual triage first. It has also vastly increased access, now that everyone has coverage, we can get the patient to the right provider at the right time."

The young physician added, "By the way, we have finally gotten over our guild mentality when it comes to advanced practitioners, doctors of nursing practice, physician assistants, etc. My generation of physicians threatened to stop paying dues to any society that was still engaged in that feudal mentality of physician protection by denying qualified practitioners the ability to practice primary, and especially rural, care."

The board chair joined in, "It has also spawned new job opportunities. There are several "NATIONAL ACADEMIC CENTERS FOR TELE-HEALTH" with training certificate programs for staff and providers utilizing care pathways with developed and changing protocols, whereby communication and other skills are taught and monitored through simulation centers."

Our astrophysicist, who had been mostly silent during this discussion of the wild ride that had occurred between industry and academics,

---

* See www.metahealthcritic.com

providers, and patients, added this. "Many of you in the academic health center world even learn to look at former competitors as partners. It had been obvious to industry for decades that universities and health systems needed to stop seeing each other as competitive threats. Working with industry, there were a few pioneers who got over their parochial bickering and created pioneer supercenters of innovation that made it easier for pharma and other industries to test new products, apps, and technologies on a solid patient base without the bureaucracy and fragmentation that existed in your time."

The 2016 dean chimed in, "We tried to do that but got caught up in institutional review board [IRB] issues and local competitive instincts, not to mention the legal reviews. It was just too damn difficult."

The board chair interrupted, "It actually was never that difficult—your own rules and bureaucracy made it that way. If you look at the legal documents surrounding most IRBs or innovation centers within universities, the wording is near identical, but the individual lawyers protect their version like it's the Magna Carta. Just like people told me we could never get rid of car dealerships and make a car buying experience fun, a few of you decided that competing with the hospital or university across the street wasn't that fun. Philadelphia, for example, which had always been blessed with 'eds and meds' galore but had always had the reputation of each entity not playing well in the sandbox together, reversed that trend and created a regional consortium for clinical research, experimental therapeutics centers, advanced bio-manufacturing centers, and centralized repositories for patient data."

"So let me get this straight," continued the insurance exec, who actually had spent a fair amount of time in the City of Brotherly Love. "PENN, TEMPLE, DREXEL, JEFF, VILLANOVA, LEHIGH—all those places stopped fighting and started holding hands."

"Not quite," the virtual **Mr. Goodwrench*** continued. "They still competed in certain areas, but by cooperating in these new markets around emerging health professions and innovation supersites, they be-

---

* Mr Goodwrench: a famous mechanic in ads for GENERAL MOTORS. GM declared Mr. Goodwrench legally dead in 2010.

came the 2020 version of the research triangle or the 1990s version of Silicon Valley. It was an easy ride. Sort of like a rocket ship. Once you get through the 'g's of leaving the atmosphere, space is fun and easy."

"Oh, and by the way," interrupted Doc Well. "**Elon Musk** was right. Space travel is now easy and affordable."

"Back to my point," the trustee continued. "There were a lot of 'g's and noise when the hyper-competition model among health systems and universities began to get disrupted and some faculty and administrators who wanted to hang on to the old model left, but once the 'coopetition' model took hold and new sources of revenue came in, everyone wanted to join, and other cities started to emulate what was going on in Philly.

"The bottom line is that by 2018, those systems that had partnered with patients and embraced these technologies had reduced length of stays, improved patient satisfaction, decreased readmissions, and increased engagement of referring physicians at the time of discharge."

"The others?" The question had barely left the 2016 patient advocate's lips when she already knew the answer.

"The others? Well, you remember the dinosaurs?" Doc Well said with a slightly sardonic smile.

"Wow, I'm digging this future," said the primary care provider.

"I'm all in," said the neurosurgeon.

Even the insurance executive agreed, "It seems like there will be vast opportunities to partner among providers, patients, and insurers in this optimistic future. Let's go back and get started."

"Not so fast," said the astrophysicist. "Before you get too excited, I promised you I would quickly show you the alternate future where nothing changed."

And visions started swirling in my brain just as the room swirled and we were transported to a very different 2026.

In this alt-2026, everything in the consumer world had reverted to how healthcare ran in 2016.

Alt-UBER made you fill out the same forms before you ordered a ride each time?

The alt-AMEX sent you undecipherable bills?

The alt-GMAIL would not let you communicate with anyone unless you had the same computer?

It was like a bad dream.

We looked at each other, and we all made a commitment that when we returned, we did not want to live in that alt-universe and would do whatever it took to live in the cool future where healthcare runs like the best of the consumer-centric startups.

Changes 2016–2026

What's Changed the Most in Industry–Healthcare and Industry–Academic Partnerships in 2026?

1. Pharma and medical device companies increasingly look for clinical research supersites to partner with as opposed to concentrating on individual academic medical centers.

2. Tech transfer for academic entities has moved from traditional spin-ins, in which inside innovation is licensed to outside partners for further development and commercialization and traditional, and spin-outs, with traditional vendor–vendee relationships, to health mix spaces whereby innovation pillars of the university form creative partnerships with pharma, Xtech (biotech, medtech, mechtech, etc.), and data/analytic partners.

3. Retailers such as WALGREENS, WALMART, and TARGET have significantly increased their health-related offerings each year for the last eight years leading the movement to preventive and ambulatory care.

What Happened in 2016 That Led to the Transformation?

1. Congress passed legislation allowing Medicare to negotiate drug pricing consistent with most other country's government-paid systems.

2. Pharmacy chains and retailers became increasingly aggressive in partnering with providers around unscheduled care, beginning with WALGREENS, and ADVOCATE in Chicago announcing a plan in which ADVOCATE would own and operate the almost sixty

healthcare clinics at WALGREENS stores and have them branded as ADVOCATE clinics.

3. Four regional clinical research and innovation supersites around the United States became the preferred vehicle for everything from start-up apps to Alzheimer vaccines from big pharma, beginning a wave of coopetition models whereby competitive academic medical centers collaborate to reduce fragmentation and bureaucracy and increase enrollment.

CHAPTER 21

Back to Blaming

Even before the vapor hit, I could have looked in the mirror [as an insurer] and recognized that if all I did was act as a middleman between the employer and provider, then we have no reason to exist. What we are capable of and what hit me like a thunderbolt after the blackout, is our need to partner with providers and patients and employers in any way possible and share what we do best, which is store, analyze, and act on data. . . . [W]e had one project with a large academic medical center and a sports predictive modeling entity to see if we could leverage our data, the provider's clinical knowledge, and the analytics experts' math and predictive modeling knowledge. Rather than hiding our inefficiencies, or negotiating around a failed model, how can we work together to provide higher-quality care at a lower cost in a way that is much more transparent to patients and employers?

The way back from the alt-universe (the one where service, technology, and customization had missed the consumer revolution, just as healthcare has in 2016) created some interesting moments. Because for that brief moment, the participants were no longer affected by the BNB (the blackout–no blame) mentality, and they started to go after one of their own. Not surprisingly, it was the health insurance executive. Also, not surprisingly, he held his own even without the aid of supernatural or science fiction guides.

It started with a simple accusation from the patient advocate. "You prop up your profits and share price by denying care, paying less than cost, shutting out providers based on economic credentialing, and re-fusing to allow patients access to expensive medications."

The business leader chimed in, "You call yourselves payors, but we, the employers are the payors. There really are only three groups of payors—employers, the government, and individuals. You guys are more like distributors!"

Wow! This would have been a long and fruitless conference without the supernatural chill pill of the BNB.

"Actually," the Senator added. "The U.S. government pays a greater portion of the healthcare dollar than any developed country in the world. We are the real payors!"

"And where does your money come from—the taxpayers!" exclaimed one of the other business leaders.

"The whole situation can be explained by this: insurance companies take 8 percent of premiums for admin costs, 6 percent for profits, and the remaining 86 percent is actually spent on patient care. You know what they call that 86 percent actually spent on patients? They call it the 'medical loss ratio,' and their whole business model is based on minimizing it. How can we have a working health system with this situation?" the primary care provider added. The frustration was clearly mounting.

The pharma executive and neurosurgeon in unison could not wait to pile on, but before they could even get a word in (which, given the prices charged by large pharma companies and the fee for volume practices of medical specialists, would have evoked images of pots calling kettles black), the insurance executive virtually cut them off at the knees.

It turned out that what he wanted was collaboration and what made him angry was the scapegoating and the refusal of so many health systems to be willing to have creative discussions and plan together with those entrusted with paying for care.

"You think I don't know what's wrong?" he said. "We actually see what's wrong better than many of you. Our system as a whole doesn't work to provide for the healthcare needs of the broader population, nor the intersection of physical and mental preventive care."

"Here is the answer," he said. "Creative partnerships. We need to see much more data analysis to permit new partnerships between health plans and providers. We can use the expertise and rich data in disease management residing in health plans, with the deep clinical knowledge of clinicians. We need a seamless relationship."

He turned to the patient advocate and put a reassuring hand on her shoulder.

"I get that you're angry and we are the easy targets," he mused. "No one wants to dislike their doctor, you have other things to complain about as it relates to your employer, and the pharma companies are too big and diffuse to get at. And we are faceless beings that send you co-pay bills and payment denials.

"So we need to start with you, with the patient's role. We need to make you active participants. Data must follow patients and be structured to allow their participation. Most of what affects a patient's health doesn't happen in the doctor's office. Most of what happens to the patient happens at home. Hospitals focus on beds, their very expensive profitable sick beds. We need to work together to keep you healthy and at home in *your* bed."

"If it's that easy, why haven't we done it in 2016?" the small business employer asked, not at all sarcastically.

"I'm sorry to say that, today, American healthcare is financially out of control. We all created that. Not just insurance, or Congress, or medicine. If you want a revolution, truly address access fully and completely," the insurer said in a calm (nonrevolutionary) tone.

"We need collaborative relationships in the system that benefit the patient. That's how we can create value-added care that addresses quality and cost. That means care must be affordable. Today, it is financially unsustainable," he emphasized.

That pesky iron triangle again: access, cost, and quality.

Need to get out of this alt-universe (actually the universe all of you reading this book are currently in!).

"But I have to give you a warning," the insurer concluded. "Most industries are transformed by people who have vision. In the absence of that leadership, the system fails to rise. Only leadership can take the vision forward. The vision needs to be one where quality and efficiency are a given. The auto industry did it; the manufacturing industry did it. We have not committed to being high-reliability organizations."

And then it went dark.

CHAPTER 22

Of Payors, the Patriots, and Polaris Submarines

Then it went dark. Not blackout dark, but someplace with clearly no sunlight, like the dark side of the moon, or **20,000 Leagues Under the Sea.***

"Bingo," said a voice as fluorescent lights shot on, and there we were in the bowels of a nuclear submarine.

The very fit gentleman who was clearly the commander of the sub stated the obvious. "You might be wondering what you are doing in the bowels of a nuclear submarine."

I was certainly puzzled.

"Well, your guides have informed me that as you passed through the bad alt-universe future, you were getting into a bit of a tiff among providers, patients, and insurers about who's to blame as it relates to cost, access, and quality. I am here to argue that the key piece to the puzzle is what other high-reliability organizations have learned. It's all about consistent, validated, no tolerance, zero defect quality. Period," an equally distinguished woman standing next to the nuclear sub commander emphasized.

"We get it," explained the health system CMO, "we exist in an HRO just as you do."

He apparently wanted to make sure that everyone knew that he was familiar enough with high-reliability organizations that he could use the more colloquial abbreviation!

---

* *20,000 Leagues Under the Sea*: a classic science fiction novel published by Jules Verne in 1870.

And out of nowhere, from the back of our group, a voice from an individual who had been quiet to this point, spoke up. He was the CEO of a large energy company and was quite soft spoken—an exceptionally difficult problem in a submarine with lots of radar noises, beeps, and all sorts of even scarier booms.

"I have been listening very intently to your incredible conversations over these past two days. I would like to share with you that my original career was that of service in the U.S. Navy as a nuclear engineer following graduation from the Naval Academy. I had the honor of working closely for a time with **Admiral Hyman Rickover**, who was a most forceful yet nurturing leader. The admiral left me with quite a few lessons in leadership, which clearly you have been slow to pick up on in healthcare."

He continued. "The admiral would have loved the blackout–no blame conference because he used to say, 'Free discussion requires an atmosphere unembarrassed by any suggestion of authority or respect'— sort of what has happened to us with some supernatural help."

The CMO was persistent, "We've had some successes in healthcare."

The soft-spoken CEO countered, "But many more failures. That gives us many opportunities when we leave this conference to fundamentally change how we partner to look at quality. If we do that, frankly, many of the cost and access issues as well as the blame game will change dramatically. Admiral Rickover would also say, 'success teaches us nothing; only failure teaches,' so we've got a lot of learning to do."

"Well great," the neurosurgeon said half-kiddingly. "Keep going. What else did Admiral Rick have to say?"

The CEO smiled, "He also told us to respect even small amounts of radiation. Good advice but not as applicable to healthcare!"

"You obviously haven't hung out with some of our physicians, even small doses can cause a pretty bad burn!" the health system CEO said to break the tension.

The former naval officer continued, "I have spent my career in high-risk industries—the nuclear Navy and now a company that produces power in multiple ways: coal, natural gas, and nuclear power. We run the nuclear Navy and the power industry day in and day out with dangerous accidents being extraordinarily rare. Healthcare cannot make these same claims. Even allowing for the relative uniqueness of every patient, healthcare is far more 'risky' than we should accept. It would be wrong for us to conclude our retreat without clear articulation for our commitment; as providers, payors, employers, and government but, most importantly, as patients and families, that patient safety will be a core foundational element of our transformed healthcare system. Indeed, we could not suggest that we are transformed if we do not declare 'patient safety' as *the* core value of healthcare and the elimination of harm as a daily goal."

Now the discussion was really getting *radioactive*.

"Fee-for-service medicine and misaligned incentives impede that drive to quality. It is incredible that, in the United States, we have this payment system and people do not realize it is the problem. If you pay people to do things, they will do those things. Doctors are not bad people, but they are not different from lawyers, accountants, et cetera. If you pay them to do more, they will do more. The whole system is, by common sense, totally ridiculous. The economic reality is that fee-for-service will never work." The health system CMO stated what seemed obvious. "To paraphrase **Upton Sinclair**, it is difficult to get a man to understand something when his salary depends on him not understanding it."

The patient advocate dug in. "I don't know Upton but I do know this. If you get paid to do crap, you do crap. It's just human nature."

The sub commander laughed. "Bingo!"

Apparently that was the only word that he was prepared to say.

The energy CEO got us back on track. "So, in this new environment, I am ready to take the first look in the mirror. We as private-sector leaders need to push the transformation of quality by creating coalitions that motivate ecosystems to achieve the same quality goal."

"So what is that goal?" the health system CEO shot back.

The nuclear sub commander interjected. Apparently he did have more words in his vocabulary. "You folks started off talking about high-reliability organizations. Aviation, the nuclear industry, even some manufacturing entities achieve that goal. But first, it must be defined.

To us, a high-reliability organization, or as my doc friend over here said, an HRO, is one that has succeeded in avoiding catastrophes in an environment where normal accidents can be expected due to risk factors and complexity."

The soft-spoken CEO and the nuclear sub commander were sending the group a powerful, and correct message, that would have been taken defensively by just about everyone in any environment other than our post–blackout–no blame nuclear sub situation we found ourselves in.

But in this situation, it was all taken as part of the transformative goal. The health system CMO agreed. "While the notion of patient safety—virtually unheard of before 1999, when the Institute of Medicine published its watershed report 'To Err Is Human'—most healthcare organizations had subsequently paid varying degrees of attention to the topic, from intense focus to much less so. Progress has been made, such as reductions in hospital-acquired infections previously believed inevitable, but progress was slow and patients were regularly being harmed, resulting in both patient as well as caregiver emotional injury. Moreover, economic pressures began to increasingly distract leadership's attention. Intense consolidation was pulling leadership and governance further and further away from the sharp end of care, and such distance increased the likelihood of blunt-end, uninformed decisions. It was becoming more and more difficult for leaders to understand that there were 'small amounts of radiation' across their systems."

"Bingo," echoed the increasingly annoying commander.

Murmurs of agreement could be heard throughout the room as the executive concurred. "Colleagues, healthcare can and must learn from other industries like nuclear power. We must insist that our healthcare systems become highly reliable, and we must make certain that the expectations are clear and the resources available."

"In a way it gets back to that whole systems thing that we had to read for homework from that professor. Quality cannot be fundamentally transformed until the system changes. And right now, the system is unsustainable," the nurse practitioner shot in.

The systems homework assignment. I almost forgot about that!

She continued, "There is fragmentation in the healthcare system that creates tension, between payers and providers, for instance. In a fee-for-service system, providers want to increase cost of care whereas health plans want to decrease cost. Government, meanwhile, has incentives that are not always aligned with the overall benefit of the system. Employers are pushed to manage something that they should not have to manage."

"Bingo," said the nuclear sub commander.

Back to that again.

"Healthcare must unconditionally embrace a culture of safety," continued our power executive and former Naval officer. "Admiral Rickover established such a culture. In the 65 years since the launch of the U.S.S. *Nautilus*, the world's first nuclear-powered submarine, the U.S. Navy has not had a single reactor accident. This is high reliability."

All in the room were silent. Clearly, we needed to and could do better. We needed to understand how we in healthcare could achieve such patient-accident-free intervals.

The amazing thing about this post-blackout conference is that people actually listened and changed their minds based on new thoughts. When's the last time *that* happened at a medical staff meeting?

The nurse practitioner kept the ball rolling, "It must begin with a culture of safety. A key element is adopting a 'just culture,' where the individual is not blamed for accidents when elements beyond the individual, generally system factors, are responsible. Accountability remains for any active role at the individual level in the accident, such as knowingly disregarding safety rules."

A medical resident trainee of our group stood and stated that "hierarchy" and "intimidation" were antithetical to a culture of patient safety as they inhibited asking for help or reporting near misses or even clear harm. A "speak up" culture is essential to further patient safety offered our one medical student, who added that, "Formal training in the emerging science of patient safety as well as quality improvement should be mandatory curricular elements that should not stop with medical school, but extend across the life span of all health professionals."

Our medical informaticist physician stood and said, "As we spend precious capital on new information systems and other technologies, a leading question is how do we use these tools to aid in the transformation of our patient safety mission?"

He continued, "We need to use all the tools at our disposal such as 'failure modes and effective analysis,'* 'fish-bone diagrams,'† and 'resiliency engineering'‡ to preclude harm reaching our patients as well as achieving greater effectiveness and efficiencies."

Everything seems so obvious when you are in a dark sub with smart people who are willing to look at themselves and others with equal eyes.

I started to think to myself, "A culture of safety must be pursued by all of us and be put forth as *the* enduring value in patient care, not simply a competing priority, by each individual in every area and at every level of our organization. 'Teams' must be stressed, transparency and openness promoted, and patients and their families invited into the process of care."

While I thought I was thinking to myself, I must have been talking out loud, because at the end of my musings, I heard a loud—

"Bingo," from the nuclear sub commander.

---

* Failure mode and effects analysis: one of the first systematic techniques for failure analysis. It was developed by reliability engineers in the late 1950s to study problems that might arise from malfunctions of military systems. An FMEA is often the first step of a system reliability study. It involves reviewing as many components, assemblies, and subsystems as possible to identify failure modes, and their causes and effects. For each component, the failure modes and their resulting effects on the rest of the system are recorded in a specific FMEA worksheet.

† Fishbone diagrams: causal diagrams created by Kaoru Ishikawa that show the causes of a specific event. Common uses are product design and quality defect prevention to identify potential factors causing an overall effect. Each cause or reason for imperfection is a source of variation. Causes are usually grouped into major categories to identify these sources of variation.

‡ Resilience engineering: looks for ways to enhance the ability at all levels of organizations to create processes that are robust yet flexible, to monitor and revise risk models, and to use resources proactively in the face of disruptions or ongoing production and economic pressures, unlike conventional risk management approaches, which are based on hindsight and emphasize error tabulation and calculation of failure probabilities.

Then a bang. Not knowing where we were going next, I thought back to Jules Verne's Captain Nemo ship, the first Nautilus. As with most of Verne's creations, it was way ahead of its time in accurately describing submarines decades ahead of reality. Just as Admiral Rickover gave birth to the "nuclear Navy" with the U.S.S. Nautilus, we were now well prepared to launch an "era 3" Nautilus that would herald an era of zero harm to our patients. What greater goal could there be to galvanize the hearts and minds of everyone in healthcare?

Changes 2016–2026

What's Changed the Most in the Arena of Patient Safety and Quality in 2026?

1. Safety in the delivery of healthcare has achieved a remarkable standard of excellence as measured by the absence of patient harm over long periods of time. Healthcare has become a "highly reliable organization."

2. Patient Safety Science and Quality Improvement Science are major curricular elements in all health professions schools and are a major component of the expected competencies of physicians acquired during residency and fellowship training.

3. Individualized drug therapies are highly advanced with the virtual elimination of "idiosyncratic" adverse drug events and high predictability of treatment efficacy.

What Happened in 2016 That Led to the Transformation?

1. Healthcare professionals understood that to improve, adoption of tools and technique from organizations outside of healthcare would be critical. Specifically, healthcare looked to high-risk industries such as nuclear power and novel aviation, which were demonstrably "accident free" over long periods of time. The "high-reliability" principles by which these industries operated were broadly and deeply embraced by healthcare. Patient safety was made *the* core value of healthcare, not one value among many.

2. Educational leadership in academia and accrediting agencies— in response to the public concern over the inertia of our medical

schools, nursing schools, and other health professions schools—
propelled the establishment of formal departments in the arena
of patient safety and quality with dedicated faculty, rigorous
curricula, and funding for research.

3. The basic science of genomics was brought into the mainstream
of healthcare innovation through partnerships between academics and the private sector, leading to striking advances in the
understanding of how "pharmacogenomics" could be brought
to the bedside.

CHAPTER 23

If Steve Jobs Ran Your Health System

App-celerated Access and Intuitive Patient Experience

*OK, so I'm into the true confessions spirit! We have run our hospitals like little fiefdoms waiting for patients to come in, charging them whatever we can get away with, and recognizing that a third party is footing the bill. If we were in the hospitality business, we would all be bankrupt. If someone came to my market, a **Steve Jobs** type, and decided to disrupt how we handle our patients and treat them like travelers who have a choice and turn our hospitals into community centers of well-being, they would corner the market. The myth that concierge service is too expensive is just that: a myth. As a hospital CEO, I will need to invest in modalities that get my brand to the patient instead of waiting for her to get to me. I have been hanging onto an unsustainable model, and I could not be more excited about using my skills to provide ways to get out to where patients are and provide a comfortable venue if they need our hospital services.*

Steve Jobs may never have intended it, but twenty years after his death, his principles on design, development, and consumer experience had spawned a net-religion, with many evangelists offering alternative interpretations of his practiced philosophies served via Steve Jobs Guidance Prophet iHolograms. I've always admired Steve Jobs—but not enough to prescribe to a religion in his name, or mine for that matter. However,

I *have* reflected on several of the resultant interpretations of his guiding principles and have recognized a common thread. Steve was all about access and experience. Steve wanted his customers to have access to APPLE products and services anytime, anywhere. And he cared so much about APPLE customers that he wanted them to have the best experience possible while purchasing, using, and enriching their lives with those products and services, from the excitement of opening a svelte new box of i-Something to feeling taken care of as if you were the King of England (yes, the monarchy still lives on) when at the Genius Bar.

Yes, here we were, no science fiction here. Just at a good old fashioned APPLE Store, replete with young "CGs (cool geeks)" all over the store.

Although iSteve, the holographic prophet and his simple and intuitive religion was not yet devised at the time that Steve was alive, the spirit of Jobs was in the room when those very two principles began to float around during the discussions on patient access and experience.

One of the CGs, a young woman with a red shirt and that self-satisfied "I know more than you do about this stuff" look that all APPLE CGs seem to wear on their sleeve, spoke calmly, but confidently.

"My contribution is simple, to draw the analogy between the atmosphere at APPLE in the early 2000s and these very topics that were very dear to him and ask that we apply them to healthcare and keep it simple and intuitive."

What transpired was the laying of a basic foundation to guide what we would do in each of our roles and the understanding that our solutions in this area would simultaneously differ depending on the communities we served and their needs. We would work collaboratively on developing foundational principles, clinical workflows, and associated technologies that would enhance access and experience and work individually to address the specific needs of our communities.

"It's a simple question," the patient advocate started, recognizing that it was neither simple nor really a question that needed an answer. "Why can't I do in healthcare what I can do in travel or hospitality?"

Some of the venture capitalists in the room had investments in travel and hospitality, and they were able to advise us as to the major disruptors that changed those industries.

So there we were, in thirty minutes creating the strategic plan for ihealthcare that had eluded us for the past thirty *years*.

I blinked, and the store turned from a traditional APPLE store full of iPads, iPhones, iMacs, and iBalls that did various things to what seemed to be an APPLE health mall.

There were stations to check your genes, and there were actual jeans that functioned as wearables to monitor "every aspect of your well-being," according to the friendly CG. There was a very cool drone section, ostensibly to monitor air quality, pick up your prescriptions and vitamins, and also do all the non-health-related things that drones do. The truth be told, my 2016 self was not exactly sure what those were.

"Welcome to the APPLE a day store," smiled the same woman who had been in the real APPLE store. There was something different about her shirt. It was still red, but . . .

It turns out the Apple on the shirt no longer had a bite in it.

She saw me staring at her shirt. I looked away.

"You've probably noticed that we no longer have a bite in the Apple," she started.

I tried to look surprised.

"That's meant to symbolize the difference between APPLE and APPLE HEALTH. At APPLE HEALTH, we want people to experience full health across every aspect of their lives. This symbolizes a ripe and healthy apple, unbitten by the vagaries and disparities of the system you left."

Wow, pretty prosaic for an APPLE employee (turns out she was a philosophy major at WELLESLEY).

And in less than ten minutes, we saw and heard it all.

Apparently, with the help of some enterprising investors in the real estate industry who somehow had the information on everybody and where they lived, there was now a nationwide system that would enable the ingestion of physician information, including biographies, license information, performance statistics, location information, delivery options (online, physical, blended), patient satisfaction measures, and interactive-multimedia-enhanced patient education, etc.

This system integrated with the open Electronic Population Health Record and enabled patients to make quick decisions based on highly relevant information with user experience enhancement features, such as filtering, data indexing for rapid searching, and connecting with personal and physician social networks to assist with decision making. Something like a realtor.com and priceline.com meets healthcare platform, which also spawned little babies. Because, for the first time in healthcare, the adults had left the room.

The WELLESLEY philosopher-APPLE salesperson-CG explained that once the framework was set for a millennial-friendly service environment, it hit the proverbial fan. Every twenty-something with a startup company was hungering to help create the new healthcare app, dashboard, platform, playlist, etc. And, as is usually the case, it was those children who made the platform even cooler.

It turns out that just like Jobs, we had started the process that created a universal access and experience delivery platform and delivered a healthcare app store that exponentially augmented the platform.

The CG went on to say, "Just like the launch of the APPLE App store in 2008 revolutionized the consumers' experience of buying iPhone apps and extended the iOS platform in ways even Steve Jobs never could have imagined, we never could have imagined that the idea of myHealth App Store tied to the myHealth Open Access Health Network and the ourHealth Electronic Population Health Record platforms would become the new norm for 2026 healthcare."

While we provided the post-blackout creative juices, kudos to the policy makers finally recognizing that open source coding was not a debate, it was a necessity.

Hospital systems have converged their disparate application development and interface development teams toward developing applications for, or that at least connected to, a common platform.

The young lady continued now in a rapid, almost robotic cadence, "A core team developed the platform itself with assistance from APPLE, GOOGLE, MICROSOFT, PRICELINE, EXPEDIA, ZILLOW, and BLACKBERRY (which has made an amazing comeback since the launch of its 3D holographic nEwhere thumboard) app store developers; application program interface (API); platform service providers and developers such as APIGEE, MULESOFT, and CA TECHNOLOGIES; and digital analytics agencies such as NEILSEN MEDIA, ADOBE ANALYTICS, ALPHABET CONTENT DISCOVERY, MICROSOFT HOLO-ANALYTICS, Qlik, IBM, ORACLE, DOMO, EDJ ANALYTICS, and others pooling their services and ingenuity to develop self-informing and organic-auto-app-enhancement analytics engines. The fact that these previously competitive organizations were willing to collaborate to create this transformation had the same logic that brought the academic medical centers from Philadelphia, Boston, and San Francisco together, a once-in-a-lifetime opportunity to define a new model for the health of the citizens of the United States of America."

"Wow, you know a lot about healthcare," our primary care doc noted.

"Yes, my father is a faculty member at MASS GENERAL, and he was laughing about the days when academic medical centers created electronic barriers to each other for proprietary research," she said in a matter-of-fact tone.

The pharma executive was curious, "That had to save billions of dollars in administrative and legal costs."

"You got it, " she said. "Pharma got tired of the fragmentation and, along with the National Institutes of Health (NIH) and medical device companies, created huge grants for those centers that would collaborate and defragment their clinical research and innovation activities. So now, if you have a clinical study to do, there is a single portal for every academic medical center in what used to be the AMTRAK corridor."

"Used to be," the pharma executive said.

"Yes," she continued, as if he had just asked what color her shirt was. "Before self-guided helicopters and unmanned drones made trains useless."

She then went on a relatively detailed soliloquy about what had actually transpired in this APPLE HEALTH revolution. It would be impossible for me to explain how the whole nerd-gasm came down for two reasons.

I am not twenty, and I have not lived my life writing code.

I didn't even have an APPLE T-shirt until after the Newton was born.

The following, though, is my attempt at providing simplified high-lights of the platform and the new healthcare access delivered through the effort of many.

There is now an intuitive access portal for multiple devices, not just mobile and human but also with entry points for the Internet and cloud of things.

"We couldn't just ignore the promise of the Internet of Things (IoT), so we made sure we provided for the future before it got there, and thank goodness we did, because, boy, did it get there quick," the philosopher-turned-CG continued.

I'll give you a taste of the conversation.

"It was nothing like **Sarah Connor** warned us about in the still-very-alive *Terminator* series (the latest release's script was jointly developed with a digital authoring engine)—at least not yet. Instead, we had IFTTT-esque (If This Then That) apps with conditional logic recipes that would confound anything but a machine and many made by machines, a car that sensed an accident, that then auto-called 911, relayed data from Health-eThings (driver and passenger health-specific eThings/sensors) built into the body of the car to the auto-responder, that then deployed services as needed to the scene while simultaneously informing and building a continuous communication channel to the nearest urgent care center or hospital selected using a decision-making algorithm that plugged into the *myHealth* Open Access Health Network and also connecting with the potential patients' families and informing/guiding them to the urgent care centers and/or hospital. (Sorry about the run-on sentence but all of that happens in about a millisecond now.)

"Much else happened simultaneously that was built iteratively using the What-if METAL-powered hypothesis testing engine. Developers further extended this patient-focused, closed-loop scenario by building parallel information processing apps that would relay incident video and sensory data from multiple cameras and environment sensors, manage traffic lights to safely enhance patient access by larger self-driven ambulances, and control first responder drones to immediately reach the scene, recruit local help, administer medication and CPR, and ensure safety at the scene.

"And while this worked seamlessly in a highly accelerated situation such as the one just described, it also worked equally well in the I-don't-care-what's-happening-in-the-background, I-just-want-it-to-work environment of consumer-driven healthcare. The myHealth Open Access Health Network could be used by humans and their caregivers—be they other humans, robot companions, or holographic prophets—to provide low-threshold, nonepisodic or episodic personal health input, proactively launch a tele-health or holographic call with haptic feedback with a provider or care team, find the best provider or network for a condition in a localized area, voluntarily submit data for population health enhancement, socially connect with support groups and individuals with similar conditions, collect health points and badges for engagement and motivation, access patient education, conduct symptom research, connect other relevant data collection devices and systems to the platform for data sharing and brokering, and even test patient health hypotheses by patients, medical practitioners, and researchers. (I'm tired just reciting that; fortunately, it's a walk in the park to our augmented intelligence colleagues!)

"The myHealth Open Access Health Network, combined with the ourHealth Electronic Population Health Record platform, and 'app-celerated' by the myHealth App Store has brought APPLE economics, fueled exponential growth, and driven inspiring healthcare solutions to solve most of our healthcare access and experience problems when combined with simultaneous clinical process and workflow efforts (including diffusion of services to automated and technology-enabled solutions) to open physical channels for access to a system previously rife with operational inefficiency and latency.

"And one more thing," she concluded.

My head was spinning with I this and I that.

"Maybe it's only karma that the iSteve hologram has now asked for API access to the myHealth Open Access Health Network's prediction algorithms to further enhance its guidance protocols. But, I prefer to think that it is just Steve getting the last virtual laugh and making sure that we really do 'think different' in healthcare!"

Changes 2016–2026

What's Changed the Most in Patient Experience and Access in 2026?

1. Ninety percent of healthcare occurs outside a doctor's office or hospital. Actually, we always knew that 90 percent of health was unrelated to doctors or hospitals, but we ran the system in a very different manner.

2. The APPLE HEALTH Store, with the fully restored apple on its cover, still has a Genius Bar and it is manned by cardiologists, dermatologists, and other specialists who are less needed given the nutrition, sunscreen, and other technologies that have made us healthier.

3. More than 50 percent of the earnings of WALGREENS, WALMART, CVS, TARGET, APPLE, GOOGLE, and others is now health related.

What Happened in 2016 That Led to the Transformation?

1. Once the Democrats and Republicans agreed on the twelve disruptors of healthcare, industry recognized a simple fact. Creating a healthcare revolution would ignite new jobs, create new sources of wealth, and decrease wasted time and expenses.

2. The "cancer moonshot of 2016," while well intentioned, created a groundswell of private-sector activity that spawned the health wearables, health drone, health app, and other industries that made government-mandated programs unnecessary in much the same way that NASA became unnecessary once the ELON MUSK, VIRGIN ROCKETS, and other private companies began to take over space travel.

3. The Millennial generation grew up and became patients.

CHAPTER 24

Death, Democracy, and
Saying No to Drugs

I have spent my career . . . questioning treatments that don't work. In any other industry, that desire for new products and treatments would be viewed positively. In healthcare, that makes me an outcast. An outcast with a huge patient population I might add, because patients *get it. When their physician is too sure of himself but a patient is still not getting control of her chronic disease, when a specialist assumes that the way it is done in other countries must be inferior, and when vitamins and nutrition are virtually ignored in education and research, we are losing great tools in working together toward a healthier community.*
—Integrative Health Provider from our conference, 2016

The doctor of the future will give no medicine, but will interest his patients in the care of the human frame, in diet, and in the cause and prevention of disease.
—Thomas Edison, 1916

Death is the ultimate democracy. What matters is what we die for.
—Ambassador Andrew Young, Timeless

Back in my room. I decided to start on some of the homework.

Systems, leadership, politics—all important, but I was way too wired (or wireless, given the Apple Store experience) to just sit in bed and read. So I did what every human on the planet has done throughout the centuries in the mid evening when they can't sleep in a hotel (sometimes with disastrous consequences!). I went down to the bar.

I was alone. But not for long. Almost immediately on either side of me the stools were filled. On my left, a good-looking, smiling for no apparent reason, fit, forty-something Asian man. On my right, a stately, bow-tied African American man who looked oh so familiar.

"Didn't you used to be **Andrew Young**?" I asked stupidly.

"Used to be, am now, and God willing will be for a few more years!" he said in a gentle manner that miraculously did not make me feel more stupid.

The smiling too much guy piped in, "Yes, he is THE Andrew Young,* ambassador, civil rights activist, and advisor to the great **Dr. Martin Luther King**."

"Did you guys come here together?" I asked.

My second stupid question in a row.

Both nodded.

"Why are you here?" I blurted.

Bingo. The trifecta of stupid questions.

Andy (he told me to call him Andy) shot in with a smile, "The same reason you are: It's too early to sleep, and all they have is *Duck Dynasty* on the TV."

"But there's another reason," he said more seriously.

"The big politics are about money, but on the street it's about race and jobs and health. You can't leave this conference and transform healthcare without confronting the single most important failure of American healthcare in 2016," he said.

I was about to say that, given the last two days, there were a lot of failures vying for that top honor.

He continued, again in a very serious tone. "This is a great country. It's been blemished by racism, war, and poverty. But perhaps our most shameful failings are the health inequities and disparities in this nation. If you leave this conference and all you do is create shiny new gadgets

---

*Conversation based on several conversations with the legendary Andy Young with Steve Klasko, paraphrased. *I'm grateful for his time, his warmth, and his wisdom.*

for the part of the population that already has access to everything they need, then all of this was a waste."

He looked at me, and with that look came a moment of clarity. He was right. Of all the things we had learned in the last two days from the wizard, our guides, the Doc, the APPLE lady, and others, this was the one issue that transcended it all. The fact that this country had created the world's most sophisticated, technologically advanced healthcare system, for a *portion* of its citizens.

He interrupted my self-loathing.

"We do not need to destroy the past; we need to learn from it," he continued. "We need a true north toward health equity."

The bartender (I forgot I was at a bar)—young, tall, and dreadlocked—impeccably asked me if I wanted a drink.

"I think I'm going to *need* one," I said.

"Before I get on that scotch you ordered, you're joking about an ideal system in America, right?" he said sounding more like a community advocate than a bartender. "Healthcare in America has been corrupted for decades by big money, just like everything else. You look under the hood at how the Affordable Care Act was built—it was built on buying off power blocks by the promise of profits. Public care and public health died in that Act."

I thought that was a tad harsh, but he was just getting started.

I really needed that drink!

"The big politics are about money," he said, "but on the street, it's about race. Do not kid yourself. If every institution in America is at war with young black men—from schools, to police, to courts, to businesses—why should we trust hospitals?"

Andrew Young, in an ambassadorial fashion, shot in. "Young man, why don't you get this poor guy a drink and then come have a seat with us and we can talk."

And the young man did both. He sat next to Ambassador Young and said, "Didn't I see you in a movie?"

Oh, how soon they forget. "Yes, probably any movie in the last thirty years about the civil rights movement," I said, hoping to break the tension.

It didn't.

"Our institutions make us unhealthy," he continued. "If a black teen is found on the street with a drug, he goes to prison, he gets sick and abused there, and then he'll never have a career. He'll never have a full-time job with health benefits. That's about health."

He stated passionately, "If a school is substandard, those children are behind for life. And then we refuse to give teenagers accurate information about birth control and reproductive health, so they do not have non-judgmental guidance and informed choice. It sets you back."

He wasn't done.

"The machine of poverty leads to treatment of the acute care instead of helping ensure a living wage. Our social problems become health problems, and we foot the bill one way or another. Our healthcare, like all our politics, is about money and power. We care less about harm. In all these areas, American policy is antithetical to health, driven by money and power: tobacco subsidies, fast food, big trucks, and GUNS."

"Everything you say is true," Dr. Young stated (he had eight honorary degrees). "But if there is one thing we learned from the civil rights movement of the 1960s, it is that it is up to us to make justice out of an unjust situation.

"So, don't get mad, get smart!"

The bartender was about to say something but thought better of it.

"We need to do for medicine what **Thomas Jefferson** did for this nation—namely, that we hold these truths to be self-evident, that everyone is created equal when it comes to health. If we start with that premise, then the politics fade.

"The whole power of the community civil rights movement was not yelling and screaming but recognizing that we were not going to finance injustice or our own oppression anymore," he added.

That was a good point. What if . . .

"What if," I started not knowing if I should say anything. "What if we made healthcare inequity and disparities the single most important cause coming out of this conference? What if the same passion you demonstrate was channeled toward not supporting doctors, hospitals, and insurers that don't utilize their resources to fundamentally reduce and eliminate inequities?"

"And," Andy continued, "what if you take the same discipline that we had to take in the 1960s going back to our communities and making sure that we were living right? What if that same passion you have demonstrated toward the wrongs that have been done to your community are also channeled toward working with your community to do the things that they control? That we can't blame white people, rich people, doctors or hospitals for. How about if we replace some ham hocks with some greens? How about if we start exercise programs in the morning that are community-wide? We recognized back in the 1960s that racism was an affliction—just as those who would perpetuate an unjust healthcare system are afflicted. So, use your economic and voting power to support the right behavior and look in the mirror at what you can do in your community to make people healthier. For most of that, you don't need a hospital or a doctor!"

The bartender, while mellowed a bit, followed, "It's hard for a young man of color to believe that after all these years of racism, an insurance executive would fight for him in Congress, as an equal with wealthy retirees."

Andy was calm but adamant, "It's cheaper and good business to keep people well than to get them sick, just as America learned that our economy had been built on the backs of those same people they oppressed. While we are nowhere near a post-race America yet, if you take my advice, the inability for a poor black man to have access to healthcare will be an historical footnote and as anachronistic as not being able to use the same restrooms as a wealthier individual."

"Oh, and one more thing," he added. "Poverty and health are inextricably linked. Government can't do it all. There is a math problem. We have a billion and a half jobs for seven billion people. If we can work together to grow our economy and create job opportunities instead of arguing about nonsense, we will alleviate some of the poverty and many of our health inequities. You show me a young black man or woman with a credit score over 700 and that person has a healthier future."

"And by the way, it's cheaper to keep people well than it is to wait until they get sick," the young Asian man on the other side of me started. "You have to be sensitive to more than the physical aspects of what the ailments are. All of America knows the impact of stress and anxiety."

I had almost forgotten about him.

"Andy and I (they were apparently friends) wanted to make sure that we got a hold of you before the conference ends about what we feel are the two most important holes still left in your post-blackout revolution. One is health disparities and inequities . . ."

I ordered another drink.

". . . and the other is the fact that we smugly believe that drugs and doing things when we are sick is the essence of health and that America's drug- and surgery-dependent mindset must be more advanced than the healing that occurs in other countries and cultures and that anything different than what we learn in American medical schools is alternative, crazy, or dangerous."

"What we need," he continued, "is an integrative medicine approach, providing wellness by healing and balancing the mind, body, and spirit—but can also help deliver a patient-centered, holistic, and digital humanistic approach to wellness.

"The system has moved away from a focus on the patient. Hospitals and the docs are in cahoots to produce money. The current insurance system makes this a numbers game where efficiency models of treating the most number of patients in the least amount of time is what is most rewarded. It's not the reason most docs went to medical school, and by and large, they hate the chess game that's forced upon them. However, they are beholden to the insurance system to survive."

He was every bit as passionate about our tunnel vision regarding integrative health as the bartender was about health inequities.

"The **Norman Rockwell*** dream of the old family doc who could spend time to care, really care, has been thwarted for most physicians. It seems impossible. However, a few have dared to venture outside the current system and make the relationship, including the financial relationship, between the doctor and the patient once again make sense. There can be compassionate care, but on the doctors' terms, and philanthropy can enhance those options. Insurance can even play a secondary

---

*Norman Rockwell: a twentieth-century American painter noted for his depictions of bucolic American culture.

role in this alternative model because patients can submit for out-of-network credits, reimbursements. Not many U.S. doctors are willing to take the risks of abandoning the insurance food supply, and not every patient is able to pay for services. Yet, the growing Integrative Medicine movement shows it is possible and, more importantly, highly successful."

I almost felt the need to defend the "great" American healthcare system, but I just took another sip of my drink.

"You won't live any longer in the USA. What are we getting out of this high price for the system? Look to Europe. American patients aren't getting the best medical advances as soon as they could. I'd look at the regulations within the industry and try to figure out if the FDA is doing what it should. In every other industry, we think globally, we look for best practices. In healthcare, we just assume superiority, and if anyone feels they have a better way, even if it has proven to be useful in promoting health, it is considered alternative."

I was going to give the "we have the best medicine in the world" argument just because I wanted to say something, but I didn't have to.

"The USA arguably has the best 'medicine' in the world, and we certainly pay the most for it," he continued. "That is, we have the latest and greatest drugs, devices, and procedures. And yet we are not even close to being the healthiest country in the world. In fact, we don't make the OECD [Organization for Economic Cooperation and Development] top-ten list for *healthy* life expectancy for men or women, not by a long shot. Countries with less technology and that spend far less money are much healthier. One thing we do have is the highest obesity and diabetes rates, we eat the worst high-calorie, nutrient poor foods, and we are the most sedentary. We take our nutritional advice from advertisements from the food industry, which is terribly under-regulated and has almost free reign to say what it wants and can adulterate the food supply in almost any way it wants. The only thing the FDA pays attention to is microbial contamination, which is not unimportant, but it's only one small aspect of the regulation needed."

"But won't new technology, the genome project, all that great personalized medicine progress, won't that help allow for a healthier community?" I asked.

"We have become completely disconnected from the fact that more than 75 percent of health after age forty has little to do with the genes we were born with but what we expose them to," he continued swatting my comment like a fly on the wall.

"How the genes express themselves has everything to do with what you eat, what you think, how well you sleep, availability of micronutrients, whether or not you're fat or thin, your social network, whether or not you pray or meditate, and whether you spend your days smiling or frowning. We are a bio-psycho-social-spiritual species, and all four of those domains affect health and wellness. Many of the ancient healing systems, such as traditional Chinese medicine or Ayurveda, knew that, and now modern science confirms it to be true. Yet, there is often push-back from conventional medical thinkers if we dare to consider the wisdom of the past.

"Andy's grandmother probably knew to tell him during his college years that if he kept on 'burning the midnight oil' he would surely get sick. But it took psychoneuroimmunology studies to prove what the wise people in our lives knew forever," he continued.

I was thinking about the old adage of what you started doing as a teenager that would make you go blind, but this didn't seem like the time for a smart-ass comment, so I tried this slightly more provocative one.

"My grandmother also used to say, if you keep worrying like that you'll give yourself cancer. I told her that was the most preposterous thing I ever heard. Is it?"

He smiled, "A few decades ago, the idea that worry and stress had any impact on cancer cell biology would be laughable to the conventional medical community. And then one day I read about it in *Nature*. Now, there are data that strongly correlate stress chemicals with accelerated tumor growth. Ancient wisdom always knew the correlation was there; in fact, they knew a lot. The problem is that not everything they thought was right, and some of it was quite wrong. Unfortunately, though, we've thrown away the baby with the bathwater and dismissed thousands of years of keen observations about health and wellness that were right on target."

Andy (I almost forgot he was there) chimed in. "My friend is right on target. I spent a fair amount of time in Africa. I saw people with HIV, AIDS before all the white people got it and we spent billions to try to cure it. There were some amazing turnarounds and cures using traditional African medicine that cost about thirty cents a pop. I saw people who were skin and bones and looked like they were on death's door—and a year later, they looked like **Serena Williams**. Those doctors didn't like to talk about it, but one of them express-mailed me some of the traditional roots, barks, and compounds. I sent it to our medical college for analysis. It turns out the active ingredients did some good and could teach us a few things. So who's the developed country again?"

The Asian man got up, smiled, and shook Andy's hand. "I believe our recent understanding of some of the mechanisms of disease and wellness, such as inflammatory processes, will allow the physician of tomorrow to be much more like the physician of yesterday, armed with the tools that range from a powerful pill to a mind-altering meditative technique."

"We can teach each other a lot and heal each other and ourselves. Everyone deserves a shot at a healthy life, it's self-evident!" Andy continued.

"Never heard it articulated better by anybody," the integrative health doc admired.

"Thank you," Andy smiled. "But my friend Martin Luther King said it best, 'of all the forms of inequality, injustice in healthcare is the most shocking and inhuman.'"

"Amen, Andy," I whispered.

Changes 2016–2026

What's Changed the Most in Overcoming Health Disparities and Inequities in 2026?

1. Access to primary care in neighborhoods through retail health centers. Access to urgent care through the telephone. Access to assistance through the television.

2. Building on the explosion of new health professions by balancing data analysis with data explanation—creating dashboards for all patients to own their health.

3. A unifying political strategy of matching government assistance with private focus on creating value for populations—paying for health.

What Happened in 2016 That Led to this Transformation?

1. Health became a major curriculum in the K–12 school system—a core curriculum of policy and change, epidemiology, and the spread of illness.

2. We taught accurate reproductive health in schools and offered non-judgmental guidance.

3. We made health a primary concern of the police and courts, and we made employment initiatives critical for institutions of health and commerce.

4. The "white coats for black lives" movement raised the consciousness of clinical students and their universities.

What's Changed the Most in the Utilization of Integrative and Global Health in the Treatment of Chronic Diseases in 2026?

1. Significantly less reliance on drugs as the solution to health. Hence, a transformation from a passive, "the doctor will give me something to fix my health" to "I will be proactive in avoiding the need for a medical intervention."

2. Technology that addresses food deserts through low-cost, innovative agriculture techniques that will provide low-income regions with nutrient dense foods.

3. Wise ancient healing methods infused into modern medicine such that:

A paradigm shift occured from treating symptoms of disease to re-establishing homeostasis which contributes to increased longevity and healthier world population from advances in anti-aging care

Evolution of advanced practice nursing in Tier One countries as gatekeepers

Vast inclusion of medical foods, botanicals, small natural molecules, and recombinant nutrients into the national formulary

Med-sim cards, carried by patients, or more recently as implants, allows all patients to have their complete medical history, along with their unique genomic and proteomic profiles, available to all healthcare providers with whom the patient chooses to share his/her data.

What Happened in 2016 That Led to the Transformation?

1. Cutting-edge research, such as seeing an antioxidant change the brain scan of a Parkinson's Disease patient on a PET-MRI, and showing the inflammatory disease behind the symptom of obesity.

2. The realization that the USA does not suffer from a genetically-mediated Lipitor deficiency; rather, our lifestyle choices have directly impacted the abysmal health status of the nation.

3. The government insisted upon better labeling of food, putting warnings on some foods *as if* they were drugs or cigarettes, and enforced guidelines about chemicals on foods and overuse of antibiotics and hormones in livestock.

4. Health technologies such as personal monitors of activity and food intake will be part of primary education.

5. Integrative health centers were financed, developed, and supported by a new generation of more globally astute consumers. These centers provided individualized patient centric integrative healthcare at the nexus of whole health.

They combined this with cutting-edge technology that became a magnet for younger people and patients, and an attractor for different kinds of people to seek careers in health, including:

- Online patient registration, scheduling, and experience feedback systems.

- Anytime, anywhere, virtual consults via tele-health systems.

- 3D simulation environments for virtual tours and procedure simulations.
- Mapping and way-finding systems for easy and guided access.
- Digital consumer experience systems that focus on gathering and delivering information, motivation, and healing to the patient via humanistic methods that enable meaningful behavior modification.
- Patient wellness data tracking, pattern-recognition, and data sharing systems.
- Enhanced patient education content including immersive simulations, interactive animations, and high-quality multi-media experiences.
- Implementing relevant technologies that enable behavior modification and that guide patients to wellness.
- Leveraging data storage, analytics, and reporting systems to inform clinical, research, academic, and business decisions.

CHAPTER 25

I Wasn't Born to Follow

Emerging Leadership
in Healthcare

2016 dawned again. Back at the conference, last day, early and the only one in the room, daydreaming.

"What a day for a daydream." The **Lovin' Spoonful** never imagined this!

There is a great moment when you are on a road trip—driving through rain and fog, difficult to see anything, hands clutched on the steering wheel, windshield wipers beating, just trying to get through the trip mile by mile. You then go through a tunnel in a mountain and come through the other side and the sun is shining, the rain has stopped, and the road is clear. There is a physical epiphany when you turn off those windshield wipers and open the windows that portends an optimistic day and trip ahead.

After spending the last two days of the conference watching people turn their minds to a different healthcare future once they got through the fog of blame and doubt, it came to me—we have been in a fog!

While healthcare has expanded light years in its provision through technology and discovery, unfortunately healthcare systems, equity, and management have been left behind. In technology terms, it would be like we went through the computing revolution but never increased our storage capacities.

It could have been the holistic science fiction characters or the fact that I turned the TV from *Duck Dynasty* to a rerun of *Dune* before I went to sleep, but my daydream quickly turned from a bucolic road trip to a science fiction metaphor.

What if someone came from another galaxy and was investigating the most illogical aspects of healthcare in the solar system? I could picture him/her/it viewing healthcare in the United States in this era and sending a report like this:

> You're not going to believe this but there is a place called USA in the Milky Way galaxy that has a healthcare system that goes something like this.
>
>> You actually get paid for doing more on someone whether it works or not; in some cases you get paid extra if you make a mistake.
>>
>> There are hospitals with large cardiac surgery units that sponsor state fairs where the chief source of nutrition is corn dogs, funnel cakes, and ice cream sundaes (don't ask me how an investigator from another galaxy would know what any of those things were, but it's a daydream!) and that often had fast food restaurants as their main cafeteria food.
>>
>> In almost every segment of this society, you need to prove that you are technically competent before you can continue doing whatever you're doing, except for humans whose job it is to operate on other humans. They just assume they are OK and able to do their job well.
>>
>> During a time in their healthcare evolution where large, complex, expensive, and inefficient hospital beds were becoming less needed and it was clear that more and more could be done as an outpatient and at home, there were hospitals still building more and more, you guessed it, complex, expensive, inefficient hospital beds.
>>
>> Oh, and get this, when it was obvious that the only way out of this mess was by retraining the physicians and changing the DNA through leadership training and culture reformation, in most cases, that was woefully underfunded and underutilized.

That woke me up, and as I rubbed my eyes, I saw that the room I was in, if it could be called a room, was white. But it couldn't be called a room. It was a whiteness. There was no up nor down, no here nor there. I looked up and there in the room I was surrounded by aliens, real, no kidding, two-headed, six-armed little guys. Green.

"You are from another planet?" I asked, perhaps the stupidest question I have ever asked.

"We are," said the two-headed green guy, "and we can see that you are disoriented from being outside the space–time continuum with which you are familiar. We live outside a physical presence you can perceive, but we have extracted a comforting image from your memory."

I passed out for a millisecond, and there I was in a spaceship that looked like a generic version of every science fiction TV show that started with "Star" with human/humanoid crewmembers.

One of them spoke to me. "Are these surroundings more consistent with your expectations? Your comfort is our pleasure."

"Who are you? And why are you quoting bad commercials?" I was clearly irritated.

"You can perceive me as the captain of any starship in any science fiction movie, but I am Ajax from the planet Climara* and I am considered an expert in many of the primitive cultures in your galaxy. I am most proud of my trivia knowledge of your planet and would enjoy talking to you about twenty-first century earth. You might say that you and your planet are my 'hobby.'"

Never having been called a hobby before, I snapped, "Why have you kidnapped me?"

"We do not kidnap, only borrow. We Climarans are gatherers of knowledge, gainers of wisdom. You were chosen because your healthcare system, while of little technological interest, is at the cusp of major transformations related to a confluence of clinical and economic factors," he/she/it continued. "My degree is in the leadership changes needed in primitive cultures during times of great disruption."

"Great, now I've gone from a hobby to a research interest," I said, realizing that sarcasm was not of particular interest to Climarans.

---

* Climarans are three-gendered aliens first encountered in *The Phantom Stethoscope*, where they borrowed a medical student and then brought her back years into the future, posing significant challenges.

"... and healthcare in the country called the United States on the third planet from the sun in your galaxy is going through the greatest disruption and the greatest need for leadership changes in the galaxy."

"We have long visited and monitored Earth, our most recent visit having been documented in **The Phantom Stethoscope**. Our monitoring of Earth in 2016 led to the discovery that this conference was indeed the nexus point for transformation of healthcare in the United States. In fact, my holo-recorder happened to pick up a communication from earlier in this conference, you may remember, it went something like this:

> *While important, changing the DNA one medical student at a time is a slow process, sort of like evolutionary biology, and the only way to speed it up is to mutate our current provider pool most of whom do not realize they need fundamental change. I gave a course on leadership, followership, and population health for a group of prominent community physicians and there were two things I heard that made me realize how far we have to go. One doc's first reaction was "I wasn't born to follow," and another, during a case study on accountable care organizations, reminded me in a very serious and somber tone that the genius of American medicine is our focus on the individual. He was proud that he viewed the world one patient at a time, he was equally proud if that made him a poor allocator of resources. We need to take a SWAT team approach to the leadership skills that will be necessary in the new healthcare—who we need to inject with this knowledge first and what new jobs and leaders will emerge in different health professions.*

Just then, two very different looking humanoids introduced themselves as **Apollo** and **Selene**. They claimed to be space travelers and they were accompanied by an android (I never would have known that was the case as she looked extremely human, but the humanoids introduced her as the android) named **Quam.**

Apollo started, "We are here to tell you everything you need to know so that you can get started on this healthcare transformation thing."

Selene interrupted, "Look we have investigated this, and we have found this group and time is the nexus in the time–space continuum that will determine whether American healthcare truly transforms, so let's just talk to this guy and give him some of the tools they will need."

Apollo smiled and said, "Good idea. It all gets down to the 'who' and 'what.'

"So lets start with the 'who.' Every planet we have visited recognizes that process drives culture and building a performance culture requires leadership development, mentoring, and succession planning. While there has been increasing interest in leadership training for physicians as well as academic leaders, you American healthcare professionals are not even targeting the people who will lead the cultural transformation. There is an almost uncannily consistent distribution of faculty/medical staff and their attitude toward the organization's leadership that you have ignored.

"In round terms, the computer tells me, there is a mean of 20 percent of the medical staff who consistently and vocally support the leadership, 15 percent who represent a very vocal minority of naysayers, and a relatively silent but very important majority, to use a term from a former infamous leader of this country, among the rest of the medical staff."

The android couldn't help himself. "Actually, 21.112 percent of supporters, the naysayers represent 14.87156 . . ."

"Thank you for that correction," Apollo smiled and continued.

"In these organizations, we found that the CMOs/deans spent much of their time on the "converted," way too much time frustrating themselves trying to "heal" the disenfranchised, and the least amount of time on the segment that can make the largest impact on cultural transformation, the nearly silent majority. If you can get to them, you can change the culture of the organization."

Another traveler appeared, claiming to be a physician. He elaborated, "So to put this in medical terms, you need to make periodic visits to the healthy 20 percent, put the disenfranchised who will never change into administrative hospice, and save your intensive care for the emerging leader middle group."

Apollo, who seemed the most willing to put things in bold terms, set the stage for the "what."

"The transformation of any healthcare organization starts with changing the leadership culture, one leader and potential leader at a time. You can only accelerate the vision of the organization by transforming the leadership DNA at all levels within the organization. The goal is to develop leaders through a systematic succession planning and talent management process, providing the necessary skills through leadership development, removing disincentives, and shifting beliefs. In essence, you need to create a path to physician leadership development through programs designed to promote a culture of leadership excellence and success.

"All groups and organizations need leadership. In times of change, they particularly need it because in those tumultuous times, more collective DNA is up for grabs. American healthcare is at least in a rebound off the glass of financial reality and perhaps in a flat out jump ball among a multitude of stakeholders. Who gets the ball has a lot to do with what happens next. What do physicians need to do to avoid being pushed out of the play, perhaps even off the court?"

The time traveling physician stepped in.

"Excuse me, but I'm sensing some angst among the human." That was me. "Can leaders in healthcare be taught or is it innate?"

Selene responded, "Great question. So to put it another way, are leaders born or made? Are the skills pre-determined or malleable? In the case of physicians, take away the white coat and who would listen to them?"

"Well, truth be known," he continued. "Leaders are both born and made. Somewhat like crystals, each is different and the same. Leaders need to evince or evoke leadership behaviors that help people see where they should head and develop the capacity to get there."

The physician clarified, "So what you're saying Selene, is that leadership involves pointing the way and providing the means to get there or seeing into the future while organizing the present. Doing so means securing a set of behaviors."

The android leaned away from a tricorder he was viewing and said, "I have found a researcher, **Gary Yukl**,* from this century, who spoke of the behaviors necessary for leaders in industries going through cultural change. Logically and in alphabetic order, they are:

- Change-oriented behaviors such as advocating change, envisioning change, encouraging innovation, and facilitating collective learning to increase innovation, collective learning, and adaptation to external changes.

- Externally or environmentally directed behaviors such as networking, external monitoring, and representing in order to facilitate performance with behaviors that provide relevant information about outside events, get necessary resources and assistance, and promote the reputation of the work unit.

- Relationship-oriented behaviors such as supporting, developing, recognizing, and empowering to enhance member skills, the leader-member relationship, identification with the work unit or organization, and commitment to the mission.

- Task-oriented behaviors such as clarifying, planning, monitoring operations, and problem-solving, to ensure that people, equipment, and other resources are used in an efficient way to accomplish the mission of the group or organization.

The physician added, "To lead tomorrow, physicians need to metabolize what leadership without the white coat would entail. The role that a formal leader plays in any moment should depend on understanding what the situation requires be done, what leadership looks like in that situation, and his or her role in getting that leadership to happen, including stepping aside or empowering someone else to step forward. Leading amid the swirl of change requires a range of behaviors carefully matched to the situation and the people. Creative partnerships and lead-

---

* Gary Yukl is the O'Leary Professor at the SCHOOL OF BUSINESS AT SUNY, ALBANY. Gary Yukl, "Effective Leadership Behavior: What We Know and What Questions Need More Attention." *Academy of Management Perspectives*, vol. 26, n. 4. November 2012.

ing amid ambiguity are not what physicians studied in medical school. It's not what the white coat brought them . . . yesterday.

"Most of your current physician leaders—such as deans, chairs, and chiefs—did not develop in a world of service lines and profit/loss statements let alone with multiple metric dashboards, risk management, and competing public rankings. To them it's no different than being thrust into another planet. Well, adapt or perish. We take seriously a motto from the MARINE CORPS of your generation: adapt and overcome. Adaptation requires learning. And unlearning. Innate intelligence helps, but as applied to new realms and under new and changing circumstances. Failure to adapt will lead to irrelevance. Potential 'would-be' followers, including those naturally and formally positioned to follow (i.e., more junior physicians and other clinicians) will look elsewhere. Followers make leaders. They make leadership possible. Without them leadership cannot occur."

Selene added, "I'm glad you mentioned the followership issue because that is one that clearly physicians often miss as a key component to leadership."

The physician agreed, "You'd better get used to it—following, that is. Good followers look a lot like good leaders. The best leaders receive and listen to the most advice."

Apollo retorted, "One of the advantages of being a captain, Doctor, is being able to ask for advice without necessarily having to take it."

Selene took over. "I remember in my management history of the twenty-first century course reading about the importance of followership and what you needed to 'be' and 'know' from a woman named **Barbara Kellerman**.* It went something like this:

- Be informed and engaged.
- Be prepared to analyze and judge the situation, leader, and other followers.

---

* Barbara Kellerman is a professor of public leadership at Harvard University's John F. Kennedy School of Government. Barbara Kellerman, *Followership: How Followers Are Creating Change and Changing Leaders, Harvard Business Press,* 2008, 257–258.

- Be open to allies, creative partnerships, and forming coalitions, even with former enemies or competitors.
- Be prepared to be different.
- Be loyal to the group, not a single individual.
- Know the importance of timing.
- Know your options.
- Know when bad leaders are digging in.
- Know the risk of doing (or not doing) something.

Now both humanoids were on a roll. The first continued, "At the academy, I used to say, 'How do you know a good leader? They have followers!' Followers aren't a genetic type. To put it in twenty-first-century human terms, you're not either a combination of prototypical **Arnold Schwarzenegger** and **Clint Eastwood** characters or a hybrid of a sheep and a lemming. Able leaders combined with competent followers produce the phenomenon of good leadership."

Selene agreed, "Good leaders know when to follow and good followers know when to lead. They understand themselves, their abilities, and their weaknesses relative to others in their group and they understand the demands of a given situation. So, too, do followers. They carry a sense of the moment, their fit with it, the demands of leadership, and how best to get those demands met—that is, what role to play. Central to all of this is awareness—of self, of others, and of the situation. Restated, it's not just about you or some macho movie character."

The physician attempted to return the focus of the conversation back to physicians. "Why would others follow physicians into the vortex of healthcare? The time has come to equip the current physician leaders capable to lead in the times ahead, to make them leaders."

Selene interrupted, "I'm sensing that this group understands the what and who, they are in their minds asking 'how.'"

Apollo emphasized, "It will take a massive investment in physician education and succession planning to make that happen. You will need to work with others to build leadership academies that guide participants through cultural and leadership challenges in a way that builds the organization's core vision, transforming how healthcare is delivered and how health is understood in a continuum, from the environment, to the community, to the individual. To achieve this transformation, you will need to build and organize a deliberate and systematic effort to ensure leadership continuity in key positions and to encourage individual advancement. The foundation premise of top-level leadership development is that leaders are not simply born, but are created through life experiences, reflection, and learning.

"The healthcare industry may be unique in the enormity of the talent challenges that confront it. If there were ever a 'perfect storm' related to succession development and talent management, it is most acute in healthcare," the android said very logically (obviously!).

The android continued. "According to the history books, and **Allan Schweyer** of the HUMAN CAPITAL INSTITUTE, 'While it is true that the aging population restricts talent for all industries, it is only in healthcare and life sciences that it so profoundly impacts demand at the same time.' To prepare, he suggests that healthcare organizations:

- Build and maintain a strong employer brand and cooperate to build a strong brand for the industry.
- Develop strategic and ongoing succession planning and development processes.
- Create strategic recruitment plans and develop a variety of creative tools to attract top talent.
- Build effective on-boarding and mentoring programs and processes.
- Create great places to work so that the top talent will remain with healthcare organizations.
- Identify and develop leaders at all levels and dedicate the resources necessary to accomplish and sustain leadership development throughout the organization and over time.
- Communicate and manage your plan effectively.
- Reward talent with strategic employee recognition.

"You will need to merge these appropriate bold corporate best practices into your healthcare environment to confront the talent challenges that have been and will continue to be a major drive of culture change in your organization."

The android couldn't help himself. "There is a very logical progression to these changes. A good leadership development and succession planning process starts by reviewing the strategic plan of the organization and identifying what key roles are important or critical in attaining the succession plan as well as maintaining the quality of patient care for the here and now. After identifying those roles, you would define the characteristics that make a physician successful in that role. Next, you would identify the talent pool, a group of primary people (leaders) selected as having characteristics and behaviors of a high potential that exists internally or begin to recruit such talent from outside of the organization. If you've started a leadership institute for the silent majority, you can start to think about your talent graduating from there as a farm team, to put it in human terms."

"Or almost human terms in your case," the physician countered.

"That is correct doctor," the android continued and in an almost annoyed voice (for an android). "But, as usual, not helpful and not to the point.

"The point *is*," he continued, ignoring the doctor, " that assessing talent in healthcare can be accomplished through a variety of tools. The goal is to identify candidates' strengths and the gaps that exist for development purposes. Then leadership development programs help them close the gaps by offering coaching, mentoring, and training over time. Finally, offering succession planning and on-boarding services ensures a successful process."

"But that assumes you have determined what makes the ideal healthcare or physician leader.

"It sounds like it will be a real chess match, knowing what to concentrate on as a leader in a disrupted healthcare system." I felt I needed to have them remember I was still around!

The android nodded. "It's actually like three-dimensional chess. There are three boards of play for a leader in healthcare in your time period. There is no right or wrong. But it is an evolution. And captain, with all due respect, I have rarely lost to you in three-dimensional chess.

"The first level is what occurred throughout the 1990s and early 2000s. It was the same game. You played by the rules. The goal was to optimize performance. You gained advantage in the game by optimizing performance and the skill sets needed were operational.

"Advance to the second level of the chess board which is where you are now, and there are new rules. You play by setting the rules. The goal is to create advantage in a changing system. You gain advantage through increasing leverage, focus, and discipline, and the skill sets needed are predominately strategic.

"When you advance to the third level of the chess board, which is where you will need to be in the future, it's a new game and you need to create what 'could be' because there are no set rules. The goal is no longer to create advantage within the system but to create fundamental change. You gain that advantage by seizing new and different opportunities and the skill sets needed to advance to that third level are predominately visionary, creativity, passion, and flexibility."

"In fact, the few times you have beaten me in three-dimensional chess have happened on that third level because some of those visionary moves might seem, dare I say it, illogical."

Apollo smiled, "Just as some of the moves that these new healthcare leaders might have to make after this conference to transform healthcare might seem similarly illogical."

Selene added, "No CEO in your healthcare future will have the bandwidth to drive change at this scale without enabling the health system and community."

The android again, "Actually, the computer is telling me that there was a consultant's report from 2015 in which thirty-six CEOs predicted the future pretty well. In that report, they reviewed several new types of skill sets that new healthcare leaders will need to embrace:

- Start with 'Why.' The new organizations that are inspirational, successful, and stood the test of time inspired their employees through meaning and purpose.
- Agile strategy. Traditional strategic plans and 'shelf art' were grossly inadequate given the magnitude and pace of change

within the healthcare industry. Blueprints for strategic action, built upon continuous, rapid, and iterative planning processes, became the currency for the future.

- Nimble organizational structures. The two-dimensional 'organizational chart' is as anachronistic as the corner bookstore. Matrixed and flexible organizational models broke down hierarchies, inspired innovation, and streamlined and accelerated the flow of information and decision making.

- Culture. This became *the* most important determinant of who made it and who didn't. It got down to captains (or CEOs in your case) shaping the culture in a way that honored the mission and positioned employees to help transform the system."

Selene chimed in, "I believe that the mission/vision and culture changes will be the most dramatic. If your mission is just to increase NIH funding for your organization or be better than the other hospitals in your city, your culture will be non-transformative, incremental, and in some cases, parochial. If, on the other hand, your entire mission is to reimagine how healthcare is delivered, your employees and managers will feel empowered to take risks and think differently to achieve that goal. Think about our mission, 'to explore strange new worlds, to seek out new life and new civilizations, to boldly go where no one has gone before.' That defined 'why' we are out here. It defined how we led. It allowed us to seek new methods, challenge the status quo, and empower our crewmembers to take risks."

The physician smiled, "And we had a leader who had no trouble embracing new information, seeking innovation from outside the organization, expecting crewmembers (if they were going to fail) to fail "fast and cheap" and encouraged appropriate risk taking."

"When faced with the choice a famous wizard offered, between 'what is right and what is easy,' we have to do what is right. We need to challenge our teams to grow and change so they can adapt to any situation. We need to seize opportunities as they come so that we don't coast through our lives. Follow these lessons, and they'll take you on the next stage of exploration. For us it's where no one has gone before. For you, it's a whole universe of healthcare unencumbered by the way it used to be!"

As they departed, the space–time travelers vanished, they wished us safe passage.

Changes 2016–2026

What's Changed the Most in How Medical Staffs Function and How Leadership Is Taught and Developed in 2026?

1. Simulations accounted for at least 25 percent of all healthcare provider training.

2. At least one-third of healthcare provider simulation time entailed cross-discipline training with heavy emphasis on teaming and leader/follower skill development though, in part, regular and full debriefing of simulations.

3. All physicians had at least twelve hours of patient contact recorded every six months and it played back in the presence of a communication coach and a patient advisory panel.

What Happened in 2016 That Led to the Transformation?

1. We overhauled the acceptance requirements for medical school, stressing the capacity to empathize, team, and develop and utilize care algorithms.

2. All introductory courses for all healthcare providers were open to all healthcare providers.

3. Re-boarding of all physicians included at least a week spent in a non-healthcare service industry dealing with customers.

CHAPTER 26

Sugar Is Not So Sweet

Chronic Diseases, Coordination, and Communication

My esteemed and talented group looked in the collective mirror and were amazed at what we saw. While we cannot legislate health, we have done little to promote coordination among caregivers, let alone patients, when it comes to the biggest national security threat in our nation—that of obesity, diabetes, and other chronic diseases. We all share the blame for the fact that an average diabetic sees seven different doctors, none of whom talk to each other and, in many cases, act at cross-purposes. And while we cannot mandate healthy eating, we can legislate transparency so that menus have caloric and nutritional content boldly displayed. I, for one, look forward to a healthcare future where chronic diseases are first prevented and, if they occur, have coordinated, comprehensive care. We have to create a healthcare system with a capital H and a lot of C's with coordination of care across patient conditions, services, and settings over time!

"When faced with the choice of what is right and what is easy . . ." As the Climaran holograms faded away, it hit me. That's the problem in the pre-vapor healthcare world.

That was the whole problem.

We all took the easy way out. Doctors did what doctors do: Take care of sick people. Pharma executives do what they do: Discover drugs and price them accordingly. And, in some ways, patients have taken the easy way out and have allowed insurers, pharma, and physicians to control their health.

One of the patient advocates was the first to speak. "I'm grateful for the wisdom and advances of science. But it's an incomplete science. I have Type 1 diabetes and was told I could not compete in athletics, could not finish my university degree, and could not participate in stressful events like beauty pageants. I turned my anger into energy and I excelled in sports, I won Miss America, and most importantly, I not only finished a bachelor's degree, but I went on to complete my doctorate in public health."

"Wow, we have royalty in our midst," the surgeon blurted out.

"My crown has long since retired, and I don't want to be treated like royalty. I do, however, want to be treated as your healthcare *partner*. What would make it ideal is if it were clear that you and I were collaborators in my healthcare. At times, you make me feel like my questions represent a drain time from making money with the next patient."

The insurer spoke up, "That's because we have traditionally undervalued *talking* to a patient as opposed to *doing* something to a patient."

The primary care physician was next: "That's the change Obamacare was supposed to provide, but somehow it got twisted and bent into the same old thing. If I'm **Oliver Stone** doing this movie, I would look at Obamacare as a 'failed character' who nevertheless changed the plot forever."

"People and policy makers don't understand that fact. The horse is not only out of the barn, it is out on the street! Repealing the legislation won't change the fundamental transformation that our friends just showed us. And even without the ability to see the future, higher deductibles as well as the mindset of the Millennials is affecting patient behavior, and provider/system behavior will either need to transform or die. Its now about ambulatory care and compensation for doing the right thing, not how many zits you can take off that have an ICD-10 code attached."

The hospital CEO piled on, "So is it ignorance or cowardice on all our parts?"

The U.S. senator said, "Frankly, on both sides of the aisle, we've witnessed a shameful impotence on behalf of government. The Democrats are not willing to fight for a fundamental transformation, and the Republicans are fighting to maintain an unsustainable model. The easy way out again, for **President Obama** and the Democrats: we passed healthcare reform, applause please. For the Republicans: repeal Obamacare, which is popular, easy, and impossible."

The insurance executive put into words what the group was thinking, "Everyone should have some insurance and access to high-quality healthcare when they need it, no one should be denied care based on their ability to pay. That seems so obvious, who would argue."

Wow, an insurance executive channeling Andy Young!

He continued, "Then it gets down to the financial reality, and part of that is where patients come in. We are all stewards of our natural resources, of which healthcare is one."

"So what prevents this partnership between patients and providers?" asked the small business CEO.

"That's easy, patients are afraid to talk to their doctor for fear they may look stupid. They are afraid to get a second opinion through some irrational fear that their doctor will get mad," the patient continued.

A loud bang! The podium levitates and falls down. Next to it, a small, long-eared alien. Of course!

"I am a Climarian monk," the alien said. "All of us are inspired by the great Yoda, but I am not Yoda. I am Edwina, a monk of a three-gendered race. I am here to guide a different journey, much of it in your minds.

"Fear is the path to the dark side. Fear leads to anger. Anger leads to hate. Hate leads to suffering. Sad, it is that fear, anger, and hate have led the healthcare debate.

"Train yourself to let go of everything you fear to lose," this Climaran monk continued. "All are afraid at first of losing what they have. A crisis you need. A crisis you have. Your healthcare system is in the twilight zone between a system of overutilization and one of underutilization. The rules you must change. May the discourse be with you."

"Excuse me . . . didn't you mean *force*?" the insurance executive corrected.

"No, you've watched too many movies. You must unlearn what you have learned. It will take a new type of discourse to succeed. And succeed you must to defeat the dark side of non-creative healthcare in America. It's all about a different type of discussion and who has it. You as a patient need to treat your doctor as a healthcare partner, not some god. Doctors need to send signals to patients that they want to talk to them."

The OB-GYN doc among the group lit up, "You know, he's right!"

"Of course he's right, he's an alien monk!" smirked the neurosurgeon.

"No, I mean it," continued the gynecologist. "When I see a patient for a yearly exam and all I do is walk in with my white coat and talk in clinical terms, the patient is silent. I started asking her a few questions about her life. She tells me, 'My son Josh is on the tennis team, my husband just had prostate cancer surgery, I am taking some courses at the local college in art history, etc.' and I write those things down on the chart. Then next year as I walk in the room I would say, 'How's Josh doing on the tennis team, I hope your husband's feeling OK. How's the art history going—what's your favorite art genre?' That opens up a whole level of permission for her to talk to me differently. I found that patients started to talk and share things more openly because I send a signal that I care and am open to that level of conversation."

"I sense the discourse is strong in that one," the Climaran monk couldn't help himself. "But the strength of the discourse goes beyond even doctors. Because if the discourse is with you, you will recognize that you cannot learn all about health from doctors.

"Take our Miss America's example of Type 1 diabetes. Here's the typical scenario: A child has a crisis and ends up at an emergency room. There they discover she has a sky-high blood glucose. They give her insulin and send her home with instructions to see an endocrinologist.

Panicked, the parents work all day trying to find someone who will treat Type 1 diabetes—sometimes it's not easy. Finally, they see a doctor who hands them stacks of literature and insulin kits. Overwhelmed, no one in the family understands what's being said. By the second night, the child begins to feel badly again.

"Then someone says, 'You know, little Johnny down the street has diabetes. Maybe we should ask him.'

"And Johnny comes over and shows the child how to measure glucose levels and treat with insulin. This scenario plays out in chronic illnesses all life long. People learn how to cope with illness by talking to friends. More importantly, people do better coping with illnesses if they talk to friends. Now the health profession starts to see patients differently. The doctor or clinician is actually only a piece of the solution."

The Climaran monk lectured, "The dark side of paternalistic top-down healthcare clouds everything. Impossible to see, the future is. But do not underestimate the power of the 'discourse.' Words are important in signaling a patient–provider partnership. Once patients control their record, and the electronic *medical* record (provider driven) becomes the electronic *health* record (patient driven), real language shall you need to use for patients you are partnering with in controlling their chronic diseases. Edema becomes swelling when we talk to congestive heart failure patients. The patient is not a little *SOB*, she is *short of breath* during an asthma attack."

The patient continued, "This is what I need, if you'll listen to my voice, and to what I'm afraid to say. I need a beautiful orchestration of mind, spirit, and body to deal with my chronic disease. I'm grateful for the wisdom and the advances of science. But science is incomplete: The science about how my mind works and plays into my illness is not rich enough and not recognized by my provider."

She continued, controlling her sobs. "What would make it ideal is if I were a valued partner. Everything feels judgmental, that I've done something wrong. If I was authentically cared about, I would reveal more of the actual struggles that exist. We fill up the time before we get to heavy things—questions about mortality and depression are easy to mask.

"By revealing more, I would contribute more to my own well being. I would be less of a burden.

"In the future, I dream of emotional intelligence and sensitivity being seen as the pillars of understanding. But at the same time, health professionals would feel empowered by devices. We need an 'emotion meter' integrated into the little fitness meters we have today."

"Do you understand what I'm saying?" she concluded. "The monk is right. I want someone I can talk to about death. I want someone I can tell what it feels like when my child calls 911 for me when I collapsed on Christmas Day. I want you to listen when I talk about preparing my child for life without me.

"That conversation is more important now than how to administer insulin after I've done that more than 50,000 times."

"Once you start transforming the way you select and educate physicians, you will create communication teams of which the patient is part. Then the power of partnership will you appreciate in chronic patient care," the monk continued his advice. "Once the electronic health record is understandable, shared with the patient and the team, and utilizes technology to keep the patient informed and healthy, coordinated in your incentives will you be."

Our Climaran guide concluded, "And once you are all paid based on objective metrics of health, and patients, providers, and insurers share in a healthier future, then you will have achieved the real rebellion and the dark side of inefficient, unaffordable, uncoordinated, specialist-dominated healthcare will be defeated.

"The exact answer I can't give you, but you must unlearn what you have learned. You will win when you can ensure affordability by encouraging healthy competition among providers to optimize quality of care, have private-sector leaders determine the pace and means of change, and have government determine the framework within which the change occurs."

"Where are the patients in this new rebellion?" chimed in the patient advocate.

"Smart this one is. And sadly impatient," the Climaran monk chided. "Get to that, I was about to. Patients need to be rewarded for using high-quality providers who partner with them through innovative models of care. Only when patients have incentives to be a part of the solution will healthcare be more efficient and effective. They also need to expect and demand transparency. If you only let the market dictate functionality, it won't do what patients need for an optimistic future, unless patients have a real voice, which they do not."

"So, in other words make the discourse part of your equation," repeated the neurosurgeon.

"You are correct, that is indeed what I said. Only three things in life, certain are. **Darth**,* taxes, and neurosurgeons getting in the last word!"

And like that he was gone.

Changes 2016–2026

What's Changed the Most in Coordination of Care for Chronic Diseases in 2026?

1. We talk about fear. We focus all the empathy of our new teams on the grief of loss and the fear of dying, the fear of abandoning a young child.

2. We recognize that races to "cure" are important but that the mind is the real challenge for wellness. An unhealthy mind is indeed an unhealthy body.

3. We practice true integrated care, facilitated by technology from tele-health to dashboard-based health records. We have made it unnecessary for a patient with a chronic illness to see multiple physicians for care.

What Happened in 2016 That Led to the Transformation?

1. We took the advice of one of the largest developers of electronic health records and matched new professions in data with new professions in emotional understanding and trusted guidance.

---

* Darth Vader: also known as Anakin Skywalker, a fictional character and the leader of the dark side in the *Star Wars* universe. He has become the symbol for anything that you don't want to be; e.g., doctors going into administration were often considered "moving to the dark side."

2. We used MRI/PET and other technology to understand the inflammatory pathways that upset the mind, trigger obesity, and underlie major illnesses from cancer to heart disease.

3. We recognized that friends are the best medicine, and isolation is the greatest killer.

CHAPTER **27**

I Am Not Alone

A Systems Approach to Healthcare

I needed to take some of the systems approach that I brought to the airline industry and the other companies that I have run and share it with those involved in my employees' health. I need to take the same system approach that I took to increasing profits and reducing errors in my business world and not wait for the insurers, hospitals, and others to do it for me. The only way we can really make a difference is if employers, providers, and insurers work together to redesign and reengineer care processes to provide better care at a lower cost, using principles that have transformed other industries. I'll have a lot more to say about the systems approach to the new healthcare in my full report out, but simply put, by thinking of the problem in terms of the system of stakeholders, we can develop trust and end the cycle of pessimism we saw in America before 2016.

The Climaran monk Edwina was indeed gone, but he or she left a lasting message. It was clear that a few things were fundamentally changed in our collective thinking and would never allow us to look at the old way of doing healthcare again.

The senator from Colorado, who was also a physician and who had been mostly silent, was obviously moved by the monk's call to action and, in true self-reflection mode, started to lead the discussion down a different path.

"The intentions involved in healthcare reform were a step in the right direction," he started very politically. "As with any intervention, it is a big positive step to recognize the system is broken. Specifically, the transparency focus is right, the focus on quality and safety is right. The Affordable Care Act rightly tried to focus on these areas, which were critical to achieving any kind of a functioning market for healthcare. However, the solution contained in what eventually turned out to be Obamacare did not necessarily recognize the changes that the decades-old "systems" would need in what would be a complete overhaul. It's like if you have decided that you're an alcoholic and need to fundamentally transform your lifestyle, deciding to have a few less drinks a week is not going to get you there."

"Similarly, even with the 2016 version of healthcare reform, we have continued disparity between the actual cost of care to the provider, the negotiated fee paid to the payer, and the cost incurred by the consumer in the form of premiums and co-pays. These three things are often so totally divorced from each other that the consumer is totally confused and doesn't understand the actual cost of what is being provided or even if she received any value for the price she is paying, or, in some cases, even what the goal is in her healthcare "plan." For every other industry, the costs and goals are clear. There is transparency in what people are buying. There is some kind of a market-driven model. There is so much waste in our healthcare system because of the disconnect between the actual cost of healthcare and the consumer's understanding of that cost."

"We need a transformation, a radical change," the senator was speaking passionately, "that will yield a real, market-based system that is cost effective. The problem is many people view healthcare as an entitlement, which distorts the market. If people believe they are entitled to something no matter what, it is very difficult to have a market-driven approach. However, we obviously need to have a system where people who can't afford it can still get needed care. But for the majority of people who are able to pay at least a portion of their care, we need to be like any other industry and have a market-based system where people know prices and are accountable for what they buy. We need a solution that forms a system that holds *everyone* accountable. Responsibility for consumers to shop around will force the healthcare sector to become more efficient or go out of business. Government involvement is needed to regulate any market, but it is way too involved now, partly because those of us in the industry have abdicated our responsibility to change with the market."

He continued. "It took visions from our pop culture world to tell us things we already knew."

He was on a roll and started reciting some of the insights that had been gained through our alien-guided travels:

"Think values: Why before how. What is the primary directive?

Any technology must serve the primary directive AND technology can enable that primary directive as a tool to move from Blockbuster to Netflix, to get care out to where patients are.

—Language and discourse to create a partnership between patients and providers. To learn, ask. To learn more, listen.

—Creative partnerships that defragment the ridiculous barriers within hospitals based on departments and between healthcare entities by creating clinical research and innovation supersites.

—Changing the DNA of healthcare one student at a time and immediately investing in leadership and teamwork education of current healthcare providers.

—Overcoming the guild mentality that brought us "see one do one teach one" education and create real objective metrics for competence and teamwork.

—Eliminate (not mitigate) serious preventable harm and disparity of care based on race, ethnicity, gender, age, religion, and sexual orientation.

"In many ways, it was clear to all of us that we were ready to go out in the world with this new optimism, but the world won't have changed, *just us*! We would need a guide, to think differently, a "hitchhikers guide to the new galaxy of healthcare."

And that led me to think of—**Ford Prefect**,* the author of the *Hitchhiker's Guide* and an expert at explaining life, the Universe, and Everything.

Is this the real life, I thought, or is this just fantasy? But suddenly we had a new guide. A hitchhiker.

"Passed a Climaran monk on the way down. He thought you needed some help as you hitchhike your way across this unknown landscape of coordinated, creative healthcare in America. But part of the answer and the issue is that you have looked at healthcare by dividing the body into organs and your health systems into vertical silos and the global healthcare delivery enterprise into modular units. None of that makes sense as you now clearly know. Yet, that knowledge needs embedding, deep embedding into the way that you perceive and consider your world and particularly your healthcare system."

With that, he waved his arms very much like a **David Copperfield** move, but no rabbit, no light show.

Then we all noticed it at once.

The "it" was that every Android, iPhone, and iPad, which had essentially been deactivated during the whole conference post-vapor (actually only forty-eight hours) came on. The screens in unison went from blank to the cover of what seemed like a book.

The hitchhiker then asked us to close our eyes and to breathe deeply. We felt a mild twinge along our foreheads and a flood of images poured into our brains. The title was very Prefectian. "The Hospital at the End of the Universe, or, How Systems Thinking Saved the World or, How I Learned to Stop Loving the Bomb of Fragmented Healthcare Delivery."

The hitchhiker continued, "Spock may tell you to live long and prosper, but without a systems approach, 'living long' and 'prospering' may be mutually exclusive. Yoda's admonition of "Do . . . or not do . . . there is no try," is right on point, but you will leave this conference with

---

*Ford Prefect: a fictional character in Douglas Adams' *Hitchhiker's Guide to the Galaxy*. He is an experienced alien journalist and field researcher for the guide. He took his name from a popular British car from 1938–1961 because he had "mistaken the dominant life form on Earth."

knowledge born of the "I have no one to blame but myself" post-vapor mentality.

The problem is that once you leave this vapor-induced conference, you will confront systems that are mired in the past and have hardened like cement. A different type of systems thinking can enhance your consideration of macro- and micro-level system interventions by helping you to make explicit your thinking about what variables in what combination produce the outcomes that we observe.

"You've heard a lot that will allow you to become the ambassadors of a disrupted healthcare system, but you also need the base knowledge to move (really move) beyond the one-dimensional, picture-in-picture video drome regularly fed to you or the reductionist sliver of reality offered, purified of the context that really gets you the lion's share of the meaning."

Hitchhikers talk like that after centuries of crossing the galaxy using hundreds of languages.

A bit simpler.

"Systems thinking will help you to engage in focused, tough-minded consideration of complexity and to learn faster from the things you did not anticipate or what you simply got wrong.

"We will transport you back to your rooms for you to do some sleeping, thinking, downloading of systems thinking materials. Think of it as homework while sleeping," he said and faded away.

✦ ✦ ✦

Back in my room.

This time with a headache. I rubbed my forehead and noticed that there was a tiny bump. I pressed on the bump and immediately had an image of volumes of reference books flood my brain and a thought/suggestion/voice in my brain.

"Press once if you want to digest this material while sleeping. Press twice if you would like to be awake. Warning: You cannot change your mind once you begin. The process of systems thinking material downloading will take approximately six hours."

"What the hell," I thought, "this is way too strange to stay awake." I fell into the bed, pressed my new bump once and a complete treasure trove was downloaded into my brain.

I found out the next morning that all of us at the conference were learning and sleeping except for the neurosurgeon who mistakenly pressed twice and spent six hours awake soaking up **Miller's** *Open Systems*, **Senge's** *The Fifth Discipline*, **Alderfer's** *The Theory and Practice of Organizational Diagnoses,* and **Shea and Solomon's** *Leading Successful Change: 8 Keys to Success.**

What did *I* learn while sleeping?

Reader's Digest version (for those that don't remember **Marcus Welby**, *Reader's Digest* was a printed magazine with short excerpts for people too lazy to read whole stories or books). Here's what we learned:

> Why system thinking matters so much to healthcare, and how we would actually use it, why not thinking systems means heading off on a lot of false starts and dead ends as well as generating more than ample supplies of frustration and anger-driven blaming. That failure to think systems will generate emotions that can feel good even as they inhibit change.

Or in one sentence:

> Systems thinking and problem solving (or non-systems thinking and counterproductive blaming) comprised the platform on which the entire conference rests.

As **Kurt Vonnegut**† would say:

> And so it goes!

---

* People such as Talcott Parsons, Ludwig von Bertalanffy, Eric Trist and Fred Emery, Kenneth E. Boulding, William Ross Ashby, Margaret Mead, Russell Ackoff, and Salvador Minuchin all contributed to systems thinking which focus serves as a nidus for transformation. For some not so light summer reading, try Miller's *Open Systems*, Senge's *The Fifth Discipline*, Alderfer's *The Theory and Practice of Organizational Diagnoses,* and *Leading Successful Change: 8 Keys to Success.*

† Kurt Vonnegut: an American satirist, author, and science fiction writer most famous for his book *Slaughterhouse Five*. He published fourteen novels, three short story collections, five plays, and five works of non-fiction. He repeated "and so it goes" hundreds of times in his novels; it packs into three simple, world-weary words a simultaneous acceptance and dismissal of everything.

Changes 2016–2026

What's Changed the Most in How Healthcare Has Adopted a Systems Approach in 2026?

1. Aggregate citizen well-being came to be viewed as an outcome—for many, *the* outcome—used to determine the health of the United States.

2. The word "healthcare" drifted into disuse with "well-being" replacing it.

3. Dynamic program testing of all well-being policy became a pre-condition for congressional consideration, let alone legislation.

What Happened in 2016 That Led to the Transformation?

1. We stopped blaming one another and started considering how to design the healthcare system to promote citizen well-being.

2. We required all proposed changes to healthcare to begin with "I messed up healthcare by . . ."

3. We created the "you can't be serious award" for the most self-serving approach to improving healthcare.

CHAPTER 28

Of Kurzweil, Commandments, and Colonoscopy Jokes

A nd that was it! As if nothing had happened. Just as we were back in our 2016 rooms reading the last words of the *Hitchhiker's Guide to the Galaxy*, "what we simply got wrong . . . ," the phones rang in each of our rooms, and the classic, mundane, pre-mind-blowing forty-eight hours, "will you need help with your baggage?" message came up.

"Will you need help with your baggage?"

Sort of funny because, in many ways, we all felt as if we had *shed* a fair amount of baggage. The baggage of a healthcare system that had been layered with inefficiency based on a top-down approach, an unsustainable "other people's money" payment system, and a growing patient population of noninvested and incentivized (when it came to their own healthcare) humans who just accepted the "it is what it is" attitude toward American healthcare.

But that was it!

No goodbye party, no fireworks, no farewell message. Just will you need any help with your baggage?

It reminded me of that great **Eagles** song from *Hotel California*: "You can check out any time you like but you can never leave."

We may be *checked out* of this hotel, but we will never again be able to *leave* alone the system we left behind. We were indeed like hitchhikers on a road to an optimistic future of healthcare!

I promised two things at the beginning of this discussion:

1. I would explain to you how I am able to relate to you exactly what happened during the conference because I had mentioned earlier

that everyone had their memories of the details of the conference wiped clean.

2. I would explain how the Democrats and Republicans were able to adapt the learnings of this conference toward a single platform.

Well, the answer to number one is a little complicated. I said *everyone* collected their baggage and went home. That wasn't quite true.

Your humble authors decided to (or fate had us) share a taxi to the airport. Though we never quite made it to the airport. In best **Back to the Future** fashion, the taxi went up to 88 miles an hours (that, in itself, did not seem unusual, but then again this is Montana, not Manhattan), but in the time it took to say, "I should have called an UBER." We ended up in a pristine room with no furniture. The only thing in the middle of the room was a tall, rectangular, smooth thing, a monolith if you will.

No, we did not turn into "babies in a bubble."

But not unlike the end of **2001: A Space Odyssey,** an old man in a white coat did come to greet us.

Before I could contemplate any of that, the aging-by-the-minute gentleman in the white coat spoke softly, "I represent the healthcare that was—and will never be again in America."

"Because of you and your conference," he continued to age as he spoke, "I am dying. And that's a good thing. I will be replaced by a new-born baby of creative reimagined healthcare in America, and you will be the ambassadors.

"Everyone else in the conference will go home, and this will seem a dream. A very vivid dream. And they will go to their respective health-care sectors and start changing—no, transforming—what they did previously by never again being able to shift the blame to someone else. That groundswell was the beginning of the epic changes that led to the optimistic healthcare future that the "boldly go where no one has gone before" guides showed you." He was now whispering as he had aged to more than ninety years old.

"But we decided that we needed a chronicle, a memoir of what happened in 2016, not to be opened for five years, but one that will explain how the Dozen Disruptors for the Demise of the Old Healthcare came to be.* And how the Dramatically Different Democratic Discourse on a New Healthcare for America sounded remarkably like the Rather Than Repeal, Let's Reimagine a Republican Revolution in Healthcare. And how those two remarkably similar Democratic and Republican healthcare platforms in 2016 led to the demise of the vitriolic, 'I'm right and you're an anti-American schmuck' mentality of cable news."

"Simply, because the unassailable logic of the new healthcare led to a healthy debate on other issues."

I couldn't help myself. "OK, that all sounds great. Not having to listen to **Sean Hannity** or **Rachel Maddow** in the background at airports is certainly a step in the right direction, but how are we going to chronicle this plethora of mind-numbing ideas and information?"

"What are you going to do, download our brain or something?" I said in my most sarcastic tone and immediately felt bad, because, by this time, old man healthcare looked like he was about a hundred years of age and on death's doorstep.

I did muse about the fact that in the healthcare I left, some nephrologist would find a reason to extend that doorstep a bit through dialysis or some other expensive intervention.

"Exactly," he exclaimed with surprising fervor.

"Exactly what!" I now sounded confused.

"We are going to download your brain," he smiled as he died.

Or at least I think he died, he vanished.

As it turns out, **Ray Kurzweil**** was right. Back in 2000, he wrote a book entitled *The Age of Spiritual Machines* in which he posited that computers will outpace the human brain and that humans will download books directly into their brains, run off with virtual secretaries, and exist "as software," as we become more like computers and computers

---

* The concept of disruptive innovation owes a debt to Clayton Christensen. Healthcare is undergoing the greatest disruption of our lifetimes, all opportunities to innovate and transform. Clayton M. Christensen, *The Innovator's Solution: Creating and Sustaining Successful Growth. Harvard Business Press,* 2003.

** Ray Kurzweil: an American author, computer scientist, inventor, and futurist. He wrote *The Age of Spiritual Machines: When Computers Exceed Human Intelligence* in 2000.

become more like us. As part of that evolution/revolution, we will be able to download our brains and create conscious and spiritual machines. Apparently this "monolith" was one of them.

But it was no longer a monolith. It looked very human indeed and actually reminded me of one of my former WHARTON professors.

I thought to myself, "Wow, is this a good thing?

"I'd better immediately dump my shares of the company that makes ROSETTA STONE* because being able to just "upload" new languages into my brain will be a hell of a lot easier than memorizing "how do I get to the bar?" in whatever country I'm traveling.

"But it also has its down side. Having my computer download my brain with its superior processing ability means that I could become, well, irrelevant."

The computer/WHARTON professor smiled (at least I thought it was a smile).

He said, "You might be worried that you will not be needed under this scenario, but a good leader recognizes that he or she should always have five people around them who think they can do a better job than the leader. And three that are right."

Now he was really sounding like my WHARTON professor!

And it turns out good old Ray was right. In the future, you will be able to download your brain.

"So, here's the drill." The spiritual computer began. "In order to accelerate the process, we will download the events of the last forty-eight hours as your brain perceived them and allow that to become the nidus for the revolution that healthcare so sorely needs."

"OK, how exactly does this work? Is it painful?" I knew that was a stupid question, but I had asked the same thing before my colonoscopy and miraculously got the same stupid answer.

"No it won't hurt me a bit! Sorry," the machine/human continued. "My small attempt at twenty-first century medical humor."

---

* ROSETTA STONE: a granodiorite stele inscribed with a decree issued at Memphis, Egypt, in 196 BCE on behalf of King Ptolemy V. More recently, it is a company dedicated to making it simpler to learn other languages (before the technology developed in 2018 where your brain could be downloaded and the new language uploaded while you were sleeping).

"I think you're about a century off," my colleague and one of the co-authors of this book remarked.

The individual who was about to inherit my brain continued, "Kurzweil correctly understood that there is a difference between scanning the brain to understand it, in a generic fashion, and scanning a particular person's brain in order to preserve it in exact detail, for *uploading* into a computer, for example. The latter is much harder to do because it requires capturing much more detail. So, in essence, you become *software* not *hardware*, and your mortality will become a function of your ability to make frequent 'backups' of your brain."

"Wow, I can see it now," the third member of our **Musketeer** family chimed in. "Windows: the brain version. I'm sure that won't crash!"

"You (or at least your brains) will be the authors of the book that chronicles the forty-eight hours that transformed healthcare."

There it was. I became the first human brain cassette recorder. It was actually pretty painless. Yes, it did require some kick-ass hardware. My 64 gb iPhone Plus just wasn't going to do the trick.

After my brain scan by the WHARTON professor (think a combination of Vulcan mind meld and **Kreskin**-style hypnotism), he handed me a small square metal thing that looked like one of those old iPod Shuffles that held about 200 songs, but apparently, this little baby held a virtual piece of my brain—at least the piece that was inhabited since the vapor and blackout.

And he left, and all that was left in the room was the "brain shuffle" and the sets of headphones, wireless of course. Very cool looking (**Dr. Dre**, eat your heart out).

We put them on and heard what you just read. Very much like an audible reader.

We Can Fix Healthcare in America OR Decision 2016:
The Future Is Now
By **Steve Klasko** and **Greg Shea** with **Michael Hoad**
✦ ✦ ✦

So this really was planned—the vapor, the blackout, the timing. Right when American healthcare needed it the most.

The alien guides. The time-space travel. All meant for us.

And we get to be the narrators of a modern day *Canterbury Tales*. And it really all worked out.

Each of the participants left the conference with a different attitude and cajoled/urged/shamed their colleagues into thinking differently. Not just a little differently but transformative-differently, reimagining-differently, blame no one but yourself-differently.

As the Bible said, they went "forth and multiplied" until the optimistic future of healthcare and the revolution that needed to happen became inevitable.

All good except for one more problem.

My colleague and co-author (being the most practical of all of us), right as we were listening to the end of the book so articulately written by our downloaded brains, said, "Before we get done congratulating ourselves, has anyone thought about how we are going to get out of here?"

"Good question." The third member of our group added very unhelpfully. "My guess is that UBER* does not go out to one-room outposts in the middle of the solar system, and even if they did, not sure my AMERICAN EXPRESS could handle the galactic surge pricing!"

And just as we were contemplating the rest of our lives in this room with the three of us (I think we were all in agreement that writing a book was one thing, even downloading our brains together, but the rest of our lives? I don't think so), in the center of the room appeared the original monolith. But while it was solid gray on one side (in true science fiction monolith fashion), on the other side, it started out looking like a stone tablet.

On the tablet, the title: **Ten Commandments of the New Healthcare**.

That quickly faded and became a full-screen (actually full monolith), modern-font presentation with the title:

Twelve Disruptors for the Demise of the Old Future of Healthcare

And here they are, from the narrator of the *Canterbury Tales*, or more accurately like **R2D2** in *Star Wars 4* projecting the image of **Princess Leia** with the plans for the revolution:

---

*UBER: a ride-for-hire company developed in the twenty-first century that was responsible for a great deal of profanity from the lips of taxi drivers.

The Twelve Disruptors for the Demise of the Old Future of Healthcare

1. Thou shalt look at healthcare as a team sport and develop a system that is both user-friendly and delivers value.

2. Thou shalt take the volume incentive out of the payment system and put incentives in place that are aligned with optimal health outcomes.

3. Thou shalt set up your system to provide the right solution for the right patient at the right time and provide coordinated care across patient condition, services, and time.

4. Thou shalt select and educate physicians of the future as opposed to those of the past. Thou shalt never again be surprised that doctors (solely based on science GPA, multiple-choice tests, and memorizing organic chemistry formulas) are not more empathetic, communicative, and creative.

5. Thou shalt never again use the terms "see one—do one—teach one" for surgical education, and thou shalt instead use technology to ensure that every surgeon can objectively prove appropriate competence and confidence to perform the requested procedure.

6. Thou shalt learn the lessons of the now defunct BLOCKBUSTER and move healthcare from a "come to my hospital when you are sick" to a NETFLIX mindset of "getting healthcare out to where the consumer is." Thou shalt also not build new inpatient beds when it is clear that there will be disruptive influences that fundamentally decrease the need for expensive inpatient beds.

7. Thou shalt always send a patient a believable, understandable bill for services rendered in a manner that clearly states what was done, what it cost, and what the patient owes—regardless of who is paying the bill.

8. Thou shalt never use the term "alternate healthcare" for modalities used to treat chronic diseases that are utilized by patients and providers in other countries and that, in some cases, have much better results than traditional American medicine in treating said diseases.

9. Thou shalt de-fragment the application of innovation and clinical research through supersites, and thou shalt cease and desist constructing walls between institutions of non-interoperability that hamper the acceleration of research and innovation.

10. Thou shalt create an integrated, interoperable legacy electronic health record system allowing for vendor-driven patient-centric apps such that your health information is at least as integrated as your shopping information on AMAZON or your viewing information on NETFLIX.

11. Thou shalt understand systems thinking and employ said models in your attempts to redesign a healthcare system that actually makes patients and communities healthier. Only then will you be able to "break" the iron triangle of access, quality, and cost.

12. Thou shalt never again be satisfied with *any* healthcare disparities based on race, creed, religion, sexual orientation, socioeconomic status, or planet of origin.

Yes, that answers the second question I posited.

The twelve disruptors became the nidus for the *remarkably similar* platforms for the Democratic and Republican national platforms.

And the rest, as they say, is just history.

At least in a ***Back to the Future*** history kind of way.

CHAPTER **29**

Of Democrats, Disenfranchised Republicans, and *Duck Dynasty*

We did make it home. It turns out that the monolith was a multi-purpose monolith/taxi. We opened the door, got in, and each of us was transported back to our living rooms, shuffle-downloaded brain in hand. Sort of like a space-age UBER-M without the water bottles, mints, or someone opening and closing the door for you.

What I did find out during the trip is that the WHARTON professor who downloaded my brain did indeed have a sense of humor. This palm-sized shuffle held not only my downloaded brain and the contents of this book that you are holding in your hand or listening to on your headphones.

It also held a very cool playlist of downloaded music.

Yes, believe it or not, the artificial intelligence being that melded my brain created a virtual playlist.

Pressing play, I heard:

Press once for the "Mix for the 'Morrow of Medicine"
    Very **Jethro Tull**-ish

Press twice for "Ten Tunes for Transformation."
    Very **Casey Kasem**-ish

Which means spiritual machines do have a sense of humor, or at least my downloaded brain did!

I have included the playlist at the end of this book, or for those of you still in 2016, the actual songs can be accessed on SPOTIFY. Just search for the "Healthcare Mix for the Morrow of Medicine" or "Ten Tunes for Transformation" shared playlist by **Stevie Kent**.

CHAPTER 30

We Watch Sanjay Gupta
Get the Scoop

Miraculously, nothing had changed, and to our spouses and children, we had only been gone an hour.

You have to love the time–space continuum!

"Where have you been?" A very normal question when I have been gone an hour and come back looking tired and haggard.

An even more typical response. "You wouldn't believe it if I told you!"

One of the great things about being married for ten years is you can say stuff like that and get away with it.

"So what do you want to do today?" my wife asked.

"How about some *Duck Dynasty* binge watching." I said very seriously.

"Very funny!" Obviously not taking me seriously.

We put on CNN while my wife and I were deciding what to do. And there it was.

We saw **Sanjay Gupta**,* physician, journalist, news breaker, health-care policy expert—who else could have broken this story?

"Breaking News: It appears as if the Democratic National Committee and Republican National Committee have developed eerily similar platforms. This would have been hard to believe even a month ago as the

---

* Sanjay Gupta: a groundbreaking journalist and physician. He is associate chief at Grady Memorial Hospital in Atlanta and is CNN's multiple Emmy-award–winning medical correspondent. He is quoted as saying "The worst crime of all would be that a (medical) mistake happens and no one talks about it or learns from it."

bickering, mud slinging, and fear mongering had reached an all-time pitched high.

Sanjay continued, "But miraculously to most of us, they have built their platforms based on a dozen principles:

1. Team-enabled healthcare will become the standard.

2. Financial incentives will be aligned with optimal utilization and health outcomes.

3. Care will be coordinated across patient condition, services, and time.

4. Young physicians will be taught the humanism of medicine and creating doctors for the future.

5. Physicians and surgeons and their specialty societies will utilize simulators to prove technical and teamwork competence.

6. No new inpatient beds will be developed until it is clear how new technologies will disrupt hospital utilization.

7. All bills sent for healthcare services rendered from a single visit, hospitalization, or group of visits will need to be consolidated, easy to understand, and sent from a single source.

8. Especially for chronic diseases, the use of vitamin therapies, nutritional therapy, and other global or alternative procedures will be adapted into the mainstream of healthcare.

9. Any new governmental- or taxpayer-funded funds for innovation or clinical research will require more than one entity to collaborate.

10. A single, interoperable electronic health record will be adopted in a manner that is affordable and allows for independent and customized "apps" to be developed.

11. Grants will be given for the utilization of systems thinking and models successfully employed in other industries with the goal of promoting zero defects, alignment, and ease of access for patients.

12. Disparities in healthcare will be eliminated by 2020."

Sanjay did offer this one caveat, however.

"As you view the platforms, you will see that there are slight differences in wording reflective of their constituencies, but they are remarkably similar!"

Wow, who said the revolution will not be televised!

Well, that's it.

Please stay tuned for our sequel:

Healthcare Is All Fixed: It's Fair, Fun, and 'Fordable, written by All Of Us Involved in Healthcare in America.

Meanwhile Back
in the West Wing

I can't tell you how I got to see (and hear) what follows—because I'm still not sure—but here's what happened, or at least what I think happened, when Truman and Obama reconnected after the conference.

A voice declared, "Let me show you how it will be, sooner than you fear and later than you hope. The incredibly unusual word 'inalienable' and the accompanying downright weird declaration that pursuit of happiness was a right came to include 'well-being.' All Americans were, by law, to have full and equal access to support for their physical and mental well-being."

Harry Truman and **Barack Obama** stepped forward and gazed into the stream of time at a family scene occurring at some unspecified future moment. Two parents sat in a room with a late teenage youth.

PARENTS 1 AND 2: Well, your eighteenth birthday is coming up. Lots of choices to make.

CHILD: Yes indeed. Can't wait.

P2: I bet. And we can't wait for the transfer of educational debt ownership!

C: You're doing that!

P2: That's a surprise?

C: No, but I still don't like it.

P2: Welcome to the big time, kid!

P1: Speaking of choices at eighteen, hopefully, you've already made the one concerning doing eighteen shots.

C: Yeah, yeah. Not to worry. Not doing it. I have too much to live for and I need every last one of my brain cells, original and enhanced.

P1: Smart lad. Look, we're glad we have a few minutes to talk about one of those choices that you will have. It's time for the talk.

C: Are you kidding me, I think I know all about safe sex!

P1: No not that one, the talk about the decisions you have concerning your Personal Well-Being Implant (or PWI) in your left wrist and a backup in a location known only to us.

P2: It was implanted at birth and has enabled us to always know where you are and how you are doing. It also, with our permission, has allowed our choice of caregivers and life supporters and enhancers to know how you are doing and to let us know when you had a fever or when a vaccine wasn't taken just right or when, as a baby, your nap was over or your glucose levels were falling and you needed feeding. Someday, you'll get to do that with us as aging comes to require it. But that's a conversation for another day.

We have, sometimes as prescribed by law, turned various oversight functions over to you over the years. You have your own security code blacking out various activities—thank goodness! On your eighteenth birthday, the remaining oversight functions go over to you and we tell you the location of the backup implant. You also get to decide if you'd like the implants removed. If you do remove them and wish to remain an American citizen, then you have a choice of a variety of external devices. Some are government covered and some are covered by our mid-cap or Homer Simpson Donut Coverage supplement, but anything beyond that level of cost would be on you, like the blueberry platinum dental grille/nose pierce option.

P1: You know that with this system all your personal records are available to you to use as you see fit?

C: I know that! Currently, I particularly like looking at the in-utero sonogram and the images of my skull fracture.

P1: Really, the fracture?

C: Yes, I keep them with a photo of the remains of my helmet. It's a reminder about paying at least some attention to my safety and well-being and not just clicking fast-forward or pause for the various updates. By the way, I have noticed there's no delete option for the health info blasts.

P1: Well, not in your settings.

C: You mean when I'm eighteen I will get to delete them?

P1: Actually, you will also be able to block them altogether.

C: Cool!

P2: We hope you will allow at least a few through. They are customized to your health, like air quality warnings for your low-grade asthma and periodic cautions about eating any shellfish. And, as you know, your adhering to best well-living practices affect your charges.

C: 'K.

P1: KK. We'll miss knowing as much as we do about how you're doing.

C: Well, maybe I'll still let you know a little. We'll still Holo and I do know how to forward info. I'll even do some f2f* with you. Don't worry. And hey, the personal locator stays on and you get access to that as long as you don't bug me about where I am, and yes, be assured, that the "Impaired Monitor" stays on. I got it.

P2: You will also have to update who has access to what. Do you still want your coach to have your OMG† ratings as you train, for instance? And your languages teacher, your speech therapist, and your audiologist all get neurological reads pertaining to your enunciation, particularly of Mandarin. Do you want that to continue?

C: Of course. I mean, come on!

P1: Patience, this is yours. Your well-being, and your development are yours as is your health and its protection. It's a right under the Constitution now, as you know. It's also a responsibility.

C: Ah, the "R" word! We almost made it through a whole conversation without it!

P2: Too bad!

P1: You remember your trip to the trauma center for your head

---

* (f2f = face-to-face)

† (*On My Game)

injury—well, I guess you probably still don't remember most of it. I sure do!

P2: None of us had ever been in an actual hospital before. You know, nearly everything is virtual continuous monitoring, 3D printing of medical products, drone-delivered meds, and haptic or HoloSkype exams and treatment. Berni, your AI health interface, was everywhere, so your team was everywhere, too. They were there whenever the trauma team needed something and whenever we needed something. Everyone involved knew the latest news whenever they wanted. The step-down unit started the rehab and when you were ready to leave, we had everything we needed to take you home—everything from the meds to the rehab schedule (complete with Holo introduction to the physical therapist and GPS guidance to the facility) to the exo-skeleton to all the required at . . . home assistance (mechanical and personnel) that you needed. Your team, through Berni, did all that. You need to devise who you want on that team beginning when you turn 18 and then at least annually for the rest of your, hopefully, long life. It matters. It's you, baby!

P1: And you didn't have to deal with the finances, but you will. The care coordinator is the one point of contact for all of that. One bill. One person to answer all questions. One person responsible for sorting it out and, frankly, for making sure that you understand it and the coverage options available to you.

P2: You also haven't had to worry about the compensation of care providers and the people who supply them with health products. You haven't because that's all outcome based, indexed for clinical performance together with our/your personal satisfaction.

C: Got it. So, when do we do this sign over thing? I've got a lot happening, you know. Plus, there's a Galllerian group playing f2f at the Intersect.

P1: Galllerians? How can you stand that stuff?

C: You're just so limited, so MWGC!*

---

* *Milky Way Galaxy Centric*

Truman and Obama stepped back and heard the voice again:

"This will happen. And sooner than you fear but not as soon as you hope. It's in this timeline. You two (along with a little help from mortals along with trans-temporal entities) have secured it."

Truman and Obama exchanged power stares.

Truman spoke first. "I'd sure like to go back and try again to get something like this to happen during my administration. Like you, it was one of the very first challenges I tackled."

Obama nodded, saying, "Me too. I'd go back and follow my instincts, starting with getting all the negotiations on C-SPAN. Open the whole thing up. I was right and I made too many trade-offs. I lost time and probably cost lives, lots of them. I wouldn't have even needed the whole vapor thing back then."

Truman quickly added, "And if I'd gotten it done when I had the chance then you wouldn't have had to . . . and your mother would have had a different healthcare experience along with millions of others. Damn it!"

Silence.

Obama, "Yes, it's personal. But my mother wouldn't want me to trade the surety of what we just saw happening for everyone for the chance of all this happening for her. That's personal, too."

Truman's face tensed and his eyes went steely, "If you can't stand the heat, then get out of the kitchen. My legacy is my legacy."

Obama, "Things we did and didn't do."

Truman, "You know what we called that back in Missouri in my day?"

Obama, "Can't say that I do."

Truman, "Life."

Obama laughed, a deep, hearty, soul-cleansing laugh, a laugh he hadn't laughed in a seeming eternity or two. Truman's grin went ear to ear. Obama wiped his eyes and inquired, "Michelle and the kids aren't expecting me for a bit. Would you mind telling me how you pulled off the political upset of the 20th century and defeated Dewey? The full, real story."

Truman responded, "Sure, Bess won't be back quite yet, but only if you tell me how you defeated the Clintons. I mean really, why did you ever even try in the first place?"

Obama put his hand on Truman's shoulder and said simply, "Deal."

Truman leaned toward Obama, "OK then, but let's walk as we talk. I'm not sure about everyone on this temporal ark, including that fella we just heard."

The two set off and as their heads moved closer together their voices became audible only to them.

Homework—
Your Back-to-School Opportunity

Each of your authors is a teacher who has spent a lifetime in universities, often fighting to change them. As a result, we respect the thinking that underlies our history of the future. To create a no-blame, optimistic future for healthcare, we believe we have to understand and appreciate key concepts that underlie the book. First, we provide a detailed explanation of systems thinking and how it affects how we think about healthcare and might go about changing it. Systems thinking underpins the approach fictionalized in this book. Second, this is a leadership book. At all levels, the system will move thanks to leaders, and we explore leadership here. Last, we all need to tackle change—the need to move beyond tinkering to create transformation. In this section, led by EVENT attendee and professor Greg Shea, we explore each of these major concepts.

HOMEWORK ASSIGNMENT 1

What does thinking systems really look like—and why would we care?
With Bruce Gresh

The professor continued, "Yes, and the complexity of the work involved in maintaining one's health or curing a patient once they are ill, combined with the complexity of the layered and illogical healthcare *system* that has developed over the years, means that WE generate results in a way that generally protects us. Any stakeholder, any of us can point to another stakeholder or stakeholders as the cause of a specific or of a general problem and send a patient or anyone else trying to figure out the system scurrying off. We all have preconstructed escape routes at the ready.

"It's kind of like the old cartoons when someone would point a finger in opposite directions, with a simple 'they went that-away' misdirection. Just then, in any given instance, such misdirection proves decidedly less costly to a given stakeholder than trying to fix the underlying, often systemic malady.

"Eventually, resignation, exhaustion, despair, and anger come to the fore, and members of the healthcare system raise their fists as they yell to the gods, 'Can't *anybody* here fix this?'

"The answer, of course, is 'yes' the system can get fixed, but to provide a real and lasting fix will not just take anybody but all bodies, including all of us in this room, and we'll have to address the whole system, not just this or that part. The good news is that systems thinking can help here. It is not new and we're actually pretty practiced at using it in various disciplines and in computer simulations. It grows out of several disciplines dating back to the mid-twentieth century with thinkers from a wide variety of disciplines.

"They all contributed to systems thinking as a nidus for transformation. Or, you can go a different direction and look at much of **Deming**'s and **Juran**'s work on quality and its improvement in other endeavors as based upon a systems perspective, especially when diagnosing the causes of persistent and recurring quality problems.

"Systems thinkers and practitioners of systems thinking from whatever discipline tend to view events as reflective of a set of relationships among the elements of a system and generally contend that all systems (human included) have similar attributes. System realities such as feedback loops can provide various amounts of data to a system of either a positively or negatively reinforcing nature. The pieces of America's healthcare system all fit together into a generally self-reinforcing set of relationships which, taken together, stabilize the system as a whole."

He continued, "The combination of multiple (indeed a multitude) of stakeholders engaged in persistent conflict over something that matters to them produces an emotional/cognitive nexus. This nexus in turn produces a powerful error of attribution. Attribution theory, locus of control theory, and various other psychological streams of thought and research help us understand (which needs to occur before we can solve) the causes and dynamics of this nexus. All of these theories result in the fact that we view the problem from our own lens.

"Here's how it works in reality. First, we come to experience our involvement in such a complicated mess as stemming from a complexity of external forces, which results in understandable frustration. Second, we experience the involvement of other stakeholders as stemming from their inherent, even genetic, attributes. Combined, these two dynamics mean that each stakeholder (including patients) tends to experience themselves as largely blameless, their action a result of a maddening, likely broken, system even because they tend to experience others as acting in a manner indicative of their failure as professionals and as people.

"This two-part experience comes as a part of a cognitive package of disbelief, and we tend to attribute the 'how and why could or would they act the way that they do' question into an emotional package that includes frustration, even anger and rage, at our treatment at the hands of this or that healthcare actor or stakeholder. This combination of factors means that we often collude with blaming individuals (other than ourselves) for what is, in fact, a system failure. We thereby point fingers and misdirect. We collude. As **Pogo** (**Walt Kelly**) would say, "We have met the enemy, and they are us."

"It will all make sense when you download the next part into your brain."

✦ ✦ ✦

Systems comprise our world. Systems make up our bodies, our organizations, and our natural as well as manmade world. Yet, we all too often forget or consciously neglect that fact, even when we set about thinking about how to improve our world or, in the case at hand, healthcare in America. We forget or neglect in part because as **Eric Trist** said more than thirty years ago, "Collaboration at this level has not been encouraged by the competitive traditions of industrial societies ..."* To assist your going out into the world and applying what you have learned as ambassadors for the new healthcare system, we offer you three items:

---

* Eric Trist, "The Evolution of Socio-Technical Systems: A Conceptual Framework and an Action Research Program," *Issues in the Quality of Working Life,* Ontario Quality of Working Life Centre, June 1981, p. 58.

First, we offer a simple model of cost drivers in the U.S. healthcare system.

Second, we propose a way to look at technology from a systems perspective, rather than as a standalone treatment for what ails healthcare in America.

Third, we apply a systems perspective to implementing change.

To illustrate, we will use simple systems diagrams to articulate key assumptions, identify important variables, and show hypothetical relationships among variables. This approach provides a transparent way of describing cause-and-effect relationships, and it enhances our ability to communicate and test the manner in which we think about real-world systems and to evaluate our assumptions against the available empirical evidence.

By simplifying reality, these types of models help us comprehend complexity, but they also require that we omit information. This trade-off requires that we be mindful about the construction of our models, that we think carefully about what they omit, and that we test them with diverse groups of stakeholders. We'd contrast this approach to several other commonly used approaches:

- Media sound bites that omit most or all context and that emphasize behavior in one part of a complex system, often to elicit an emotional response such as anger or fear.

- Politically or ideologically driven messaging that deliberately obscures or omits important dynamics that do not fit an intended viewpoint.

- Reductionist academic research that explores one aspect of a complex issue in great detail, but that does not tie findings to broader systemic behavior in a meaningful way.

Let's start with a model that provides a whole system viewpoint of cost drivers in the U.S. healthcare system. Suppose we conceptualized America's healthcare system in terms of consumer behavior, provider and supplier behavior, and financial stakeholders. In this model, consumers receive services and products, providers and suppliers provide the services and products consumed, and financial stakeholders pay for the products and services consumed.

Obviously, such large categories or buckets lump stakeholders with something in common, but also with much that differentiates them. However, this basic grouping can help to provide an overview of that over 17 percent of America's economy that is its vast and sprawling system of healthcare. The accompanying figure presents one possible way of thinking about the relationships among consumers, providers and suppliers, and financial stakeholders, albeit a simplified one.

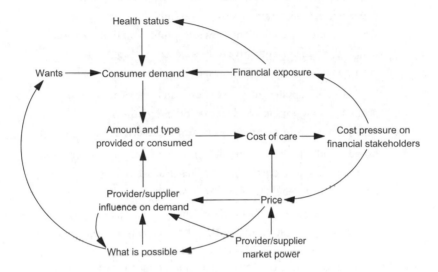

In this model, consumption of services and products is driven by the way in which consumer demand interacts with influence by providers and suppliers. Health status (which influences which services and products are needed), wants (which influence the services and products that the consumer would like to receive), and financial exposure (the amount of out-of-pocket cost that the consumer will bear) combine to drive consumer demand. Providers and suppliers influence demand by continually expanding what is possible by using market power to influence consumption and by pricing to maximize profits.

As you think about how you will be the drivers in your post-conference "checkout" into the real world, this figure will immediately suggest several tried-and-true ways for financial stakeholders to reduce cost pressure—increasing consumer financial exposure (e.g., by increased premiums, copays, and deductibles), and putting downward pressure on prices (e.g., price negotiations, government price controls, changes in the way in which the federal government pays for drugs). It also suggests that costs may be driven by several factors over which financial stakeholders have limited control (e.g., health status and provider/supplier influence on demand and respective market power).

- Innovation and the ongoing expansion of what is possible may result in better and less expensive care, but it may also produce expensive diagnostic and treatment technologies that mainly serve to increase supplier and provider profits and that may not, in fact, provide more effective or less expensive care, than do existing technologies, techniques, or pharmaceuticals.
- Providers and suppliers may drive demand for expensive (and profitable) new products and technologies by influencing consumer wants (e.g., direct-to-consumer advertising).
- Provider and supplier market power may influence prices and also shape demand in a way that maximizes profitability but that does not necessarily benefit the consumer of care.
- Health status may be influenced by consumer financial exposure by encouraging, restraining, or shaping what care is demanded.

The connections in this simple model suggest that the relief of cost pressure on financial stakeholders may require a set of coordinated and systemic interventions that influence not only consumer financial exposure and price, but also provider and supplier market power, consumer wants and knowledge, health status drivers, and, perhaps, the trajectory of technological development.

Simple models like this can serve as a powerful catalyst for change by allowing various stakeholder groups to articulate and test their ideas and assumptions about the way in which particular interventions might play out in the complex U.S. healthcare system. They can add value to strategy and policy discussions by encouraging a broad, whole-system viewpoint; creating an explicit graphic representation of the system under consideration; articulating and furthering consideration of potential feedback loops, trade-offs, unintended consequences, and stakeholder perspectives; and helping stakeholders understand the perspectives of other stakeholders.

The technology and technologic aspirations that fill our "present" world reflect an oddly retro hope—namely, that technology itself will save us. "Technology will save us from climate change, aging, chemical pollutants, overeating and under-exercising, world population growth, enemies at home and abroad, and, ultimately, even from ourselves." The 1960s and 1970s drove from the forefront the worship of the scientist of the 1950s, that white-coated purveyor of nuclear energy and a world freed of mosquitos by DDT. The religion gestated and morphed. The 1980s and 1990s saw a repackaging of fears about technology into the form of cyborgs even as implants became a regular part of medicine as did body piercing of fashion. By the twenty-first century, the religion reappeared in the form of high-tech deities and geeks as trendy along with digital and genomic technology as incomprehensible, even mysterious, saving graces.

Lost in the renewed rush to worship technology and its maven priests was the perspective that, arguably, the greatest period of technological advance in human history had long passed and had profound lessons to offer. It had occurred during the last part of the nineteenth and first part of the twentieth centuries and included previously unfathomable technological advances: electricity (including electrical machinery and infrastructure); telephony; radio; voice recording; automobiles (and vast networks of highways and bridges); airplanes (and a worldwide system of airports); refrigeration; vaccinations; the Haber-Bosch process; Bessemer steel technology; petrochemicals; heavy, civil, and chemical engineering; paper and packaging; the internal combustion engine; canned, bottled, and frozen food; worldwide analog and wireless communication; the fundamentals of radar; and the beginning of Goddard's work on liquid-fueled rockets. We may well never see such an onslaught of life-altering technology again.

What we did see following this onslaught were staggering and unanticipated consequences such as a massive, global, knee-buckling economic depression facilitated at least in part by national and international financial systems that simply could not keep up cognitively and went primitive emotionally. Not unlike "the big short of 2008." We also experienced two world wars that, combined, produced an estimated 125,000,000 or more total deaths (out of an annual world population of about 2,000,000,000), due in no small part to our technologically enhanced capacity to kill both warriors and civilians in ways not foreseen by **Pasteur, Edison, Henry Ford**, or the **Wright brothers**. Of course, a war utilizing "new" technology (i.e., nuclear, biologic, digital virus, or perhaps genomic) could easily surpass such numbers. The point here is not to promote a Luddite argument. Rather, it is to depict technology advancement as, in and of itself, neither good nor bad. A systems perspective can assist contemplation of the impact of technology even as values need to guide its application.

Technology and healthcare have fit tightly together for at least fifty years. Technologic advances have furthered medical science and clinical practice. Imaging, for instance, has advanced both information available and treatments possible. Surgery has expanded the domain of the possible by equipping surgeons with ever-more-advanced tools, up to and including robotic aides. Implants and implantable devices allow the replacement of damaged or worn-out organic parts of human systems—cardiovascular, muscular skeletal, organ, and even neurologic. Scientific advances in the capacity to understand the genome have both enhanced our knowledge and driven ways to leverage it clinically.

Technologic advances outside of medical and clinical research have fed current and anticipated medical practice alike. The Internet and high-definition imaging enable access to healthcare providers and can expedite the application of the skills of world-class specialists to cases in the remotest of locations and the collection of massive quantities of clinical data by aggregating individual clinical profiles. Miniaturization and advances in digital technology can convert a phone into a data collector, health counselor, and physician aide and a touchpad into a haptic transmitter. This type of technologic advance, in particular, has fueled a widespread rekindling of belief that technology will save us, or at least save our healthcare system. Let's step back for a moment and consider how such technology might fit in America's healthcare system.

The cost of healthcare technology is a very important driver of overall healthcare expense, and the use of expensive diagnostic and treatment technologies is greater in the United States than in other industrialized countries. In many cases, the use of these expensive technologies in the United States does not produce better outcomes or longevity.

Healthcare technology is used as a competitive lever by many providers in what is often called the medical arms race; competing providers tout their leading-edge technology to attract physicians and patients, even when the newer and much more expensive technology has not been proven to provide better outcomes—for example, proton beam therapy for prostate cancer. This set of dynamics is reinforced by a payment system that largely fails to discriminate based on cost effectiveness. The accompanying figure provides one way of thinking about how these dynamics influence the trajectory and results of technological development and the cost effectiveness (or ineffectiveness) of technology in healthcare.

In this model, the payment system—and, in particular, the extent to which payments are based on effectiveness and cost—influences health benefit per dollar of healthcare spending and also the focus of technological development (the amount of new development focused on high-value technologies).

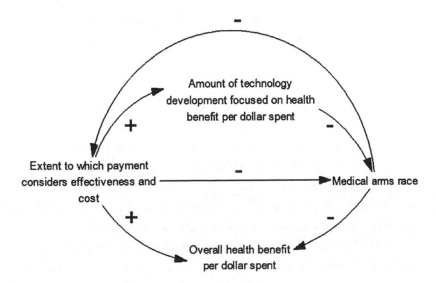

This model also provides a way of thinking about the medical arms race. In this representation, medical arms race dynamics have an inverse relationship with payments focused on effectiveness and cost for two reasons:

First, in a medical arms race, new technology is adopted quickly, in part to provide a competitive advantage; providers can claim that they have technologies that their competitors do not have. This provides a competitive incentive for providers to emphasize high-tech novelty rather than value.

Second, payments not based on effectiveness and cost provide an economic incentive for providers to produce a steady stream of new and enhanced revenue-generating services, regardless of the amount of health benefit that they provide.

These powerful competitive and economic incentives result in a set of escalation dynamics with providers attempting to leapfrog each other. In illustration form, these escalation dynamics look like this:

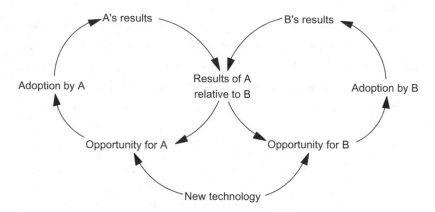

In this model, new technology emerges and is available to two competing providers, Provider A and Provider B. If Provider A takes advantage of the opportunity to adopt the technology and Provider B does not, then A's results will improve and B's will not. In a highly concentrated market like most hospital markets, A's gain will be at the expense of B, so both players view this as a zero sum game, particularly if this experience is repeated over time with many new technologies.

With these dynamics, the combination of a large and continually expanding number of new healthcare services and products—many of which do not produce a great deal of value per dollar spent with an accommodative payment system—produces a great deal of cost growth without proportional improvements in health.

These types of escalation dynamics, of course, are not unique to healthcare, but the economic consequences are, due to America's combination of third-party insurance and government payments for healthcare.

Consumers of healthcare services want the very latest technology, even though they often do not understand the potential clinical benefits or lack thereof, and they don't care a great deal about the cost when out-of-pocket costs are very limited. So, the costs of the continually growing number of low-value services get baked in to private insurance premiums and governmental payments. Ultimately, low-value technologies are subsidized by a combination of tax increases, higher government debt, and complex social trade-offs. Rapidly increasing Medicaid costs, for example, cause distress to state budgets and divert funds from education, highway, and other infrastructure projects.

Several seemingly obvious solutions to this problem are fraught with complications. Creating more financial exposure for consumers via higher copayments and deductibles, for example, involves putting many people at risk financially without providing them with a way of making good decisions because it requires them to navigate very complex, sometimes life-and-death, decisions.

The creation of a governmental mechanism, such as the NICE effort in the United Kingdom, to evaluate effectiveness and cost–benefit, would require the government to define "effectiveness" and "cost–benefit," make difficult trade-offs, and be subject to regulatory capture; it would also face withering opposition by a populace with low trust of government (remember **Sarah Palin**'s death panels!).

Ultimately, the solution may involve a delicate balance of nuanced and gradual payment changes that consider effectiveness and cost, increased consumer financial exposure combined with care navigators or advisors to help consumers with complex decisions, private- and public-sector cooperation to develop standardized methodologies for evaluating effectiveness and cost–benefit, and true transparency—available to all in a user-friendly format—of the effectiveness and cost–benefit trade-offs of new technologies.

In summary, as Trist wrote more than thirty years ago, "The on-coming information technologies, especially those concerned with the microprocessor and telecommunication, give immense scope for solving many current problems—if the right value choices can be made." Systems theory helps to articulate the choices, such as why use technology to move faster along cow paths to redesign around the patient experience? Another choice is whether the interface both between people and machines (e.g., phones) should serve to increase the connection among people in an increasingly fragmented and isolated world or contribute to their isolation and fragmentation and, thereby, contribute to the demise of the elderly and to the suicide rate of the young and old, of veterans and civilians.

So, as you leave the conference and expect to "transform and re-imagine" your organization, remember that systems comprise organizations. Sociotechnical theory prompts us to delineate those systems and to consider their impact on actual behavior. Systems deliver what they are designed to deliver. Hence, what we get tells us what the system was designed to deliver. If you want something else, then figure out what that something is. Specify it. Storyboard it. Pay attention to the details of the social reality that you wish to create because those details will matter. Then work backward to what kind of system will produce that world, that reality. If one dimension of the system, such as technology, is changing, then examine its contribution to what the system delivers as well as how, in the context of the design of the entire system and the desired outcome of that system. For example, changes might be coordinated in the one dimension (e.g., information technology) and should be coordinated with changes in other system dimensions (e.g., protocols for practice, training, decision making, and reimbursement) in order to secure desired system outcomes. Otherwise, overweighting attention to the part without consideration of the whole will waste resources by likely producing little or no change to the system. The system overwhelms the changes in the part, perhaps distorting the system in the process as other system components adjusting to neutralize the change in the one component, e.g., technology.

Michael Hammer came to a complementary conclusion following a different route, namely as one of the premier process engineering experts of his time. He wrote in 1990,* "The usual methods for boosting performance—process, rationalization, and automation—haven't yielded the dramatic improvements companies need. In particular, heavy investments in information technology have delivered disappointing results, largely because companies tend to use technology to mechanize old ways of doing business. They leave the existing processes intact and use computers simply to speed them up. It is time to stop paving the cow paths. Instead of embedding outdated processes in silicon and software, we should obliterate them and start over."

Hammer goes on to say, "Reengineering triggers changes of many kinds. Job designs, organizational structures, management systems, anything associated with the process, must be refashioned in an integrated way . . . The extent of these changes suggests one factor that is necessary for reengineering to succeed: executive leadership with real vision."

The question, then, for any leader and especially for any senior leader comes down to this: If your organization acted in accord with your vision, your strategy, then what scenes, what sets of behaviors would characterize your organization? Who would be doing what in which situation, predictably, time after time? What stories would people tell in order to capture the way your organization went about doing what it does? What would the storyboard of "the way things actually work around here" look like? Returning to traditional systems thinking about organizations, "A vision of a possible alternative mode is a necessary condition for bringing about substantial change . . . But the vision and the philosophy make little sense to most of those concerned until the process of enactment begins."† The Work Systems Model of Change advocates beginning the process of enactment by crafting the stories to characterize the organization in order to design the systems to make those stories likely to occur.

For more senior executives in particular, structure is the delivery mechanism of intent, not structure—in the narrow sense of lines and

---

* HBR, "Re-engineering Work: Don't Automate, Obliterate," July–August 1990.

† Trist, 1981, citing Weick, 1979.

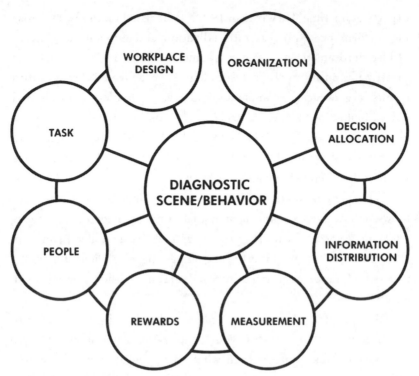

Copyright: Shea and Associates, Inc.

boxes on an organization chart—but rather structure as the set of systems that comprise the environment at work, that send the messages of where and how to focus. The book *Leading Successful Change: 8 Keys to Making Change Work,** presents the Work Systems Model, which depicts eight such systems as driving patterns behavior. Together, they comprise the environment at work to which individuals and groups adapt: organization, workplace design, task, people, rewards, measurement, information distribution, and decision allocation. These subsystems characterize an organization and produce the "at my seat" environment that drives behavior. They also amount to levers of change. Align the levers one way and one set of behaviors (perhaps a set indicative of little if any

---

* Gregory P. Shea and Cassie A. Solomon, *Leading Successful Change: 8 Keys To Making Change Work*, Wharton Digital Press.

risk taking) makes sense. Align the levers another way and another set of behaviors (perhaps a set indicative of bold if data based risk taking) makes sense.

Here is the Work System Model in graphic form.

In the following table, there are descriptions of the eight components of work systems—components which also constitute eight levels of change.

Lever	Definition
1. Organization	Structure (vertical chain of command and horizontal means of interconnection); the organizational chart; also task forces, project groups, and committees
2. Workplace design	Layout of physical and virtual space; also available, work tools and technology
3. Task	Work processes, protocols, and pathways
4. People	Selection, skills, learning, and orientation of the focal organizational, business unit, department, or work unit members
5. Rewards	Rewards and punishments of every sort germane to the desired behavior or scene; compensation; intrinsic and extrinsic rewards
6. Measurement	Metrics; scorecard of performance
7. Information distribution	Who knows what, when, and how (means and manner of being informed, e.g., push or pull)
8. Decision allocation	Who participates when, in what way, in which decisions

What then do we want healthcare patients to be: proactive managers of their own care or passive generators of revenue for other healthcare stakeholders? We can design systems to produce either. Is the electronic medical record (EMR) the point, or is the point to have a different set of people making healthcare decisions in a different way using different information (and generating different information for the use of others), all as measured and rewarded in a different manner? We can design change efforts to produce either. First, though, we should increase our awareness about the choices that we are making. Systems thinking at the very least helps to enhance that awareness.*

HOMEWORK ASSIGNMENT 2

Notes on Leadership for the Working Leader . . . and Follower

Treatments of leadership abound. They range from "let me tell you how I did it, kid" to more sophisticated versions of **Plutarch**'s "great man" studies to careful social science to case studies taken separately or in aggregate. We have learned a lot about the topic, especially since the mid-twentieth century.

Trying to use this space (and your time) to add to that bookshelf would most likely not serve anyone well. Instead, a number of key notions follow that receive less attention and rarely appear in public together. More importantly, leaders often find them helpful.

1. *How you think about leadership matters.* Leaders are people, as are followers. Leadership is a function. The function includes envisioning an end state as well as delivering followers to it. A leadership moment, as **Michael Useem** might term it, includes the demands of a situation, the needs of a group given that situation, and an individual's abilities. Effective organizations over time demonstrate the capacity to scout their environment and then to pursue a trajectory that fits it and their capacities. Effective leaders know themselves and their team members well enough to lead and to follow as appropriate.

   Implication: Concentrate on facilitating effective leadership. Continually ask yourself: (a) What does the group or organization need to understand about the world it is in or will be in? (b) What leadership does the group or organization need in order to survive, even prosper in that world? (c) How can you best help that needed leadership to occur (e.g., by leading or by following)?

2. *Leadership requires followers and effective leadership requires effective followers.* Leadership is a relationship. It requires at least one person to be influenced by another in the direction that the other is trying to influence. Absent that relationship, no leadership occurs. Leadership cannot occur in a relational vacuum. Those who think it can are (a) delusional and (b) likely headed for a very sobering time. Leadership centers on influencing others or, restated, acquiring and exerting influence over the behavior of others. That power can rest on formal position or on one's expertise, personality, or character. Successful application of that power over time turns on understanding the situation, leadership, and self. For example, it's as important over time to understand when following the lead of another will not only serve the group or organization better in the moment (e.g., that other individual or

group may carry much more expertise in how to handle a given situation than you do), but also serve to deepen others' willingness to follow your lead another time (i.e., they come to trust that you know what you don't know and act accordingly).

Implication: If you want to lead effectively over time, then work especially hard on the real "hard stuff"—namely, your relational skills generally and when to use what type of influence or power.

3. *To lead well, learn to follow well.* The two skill sets are remarkably similar; hence, to learn one helps to learn the other and, as a leader, developing good followers helps improve the leadership of the group both today and tomorrow. For instance, **Robert Kelley**, in an oft-used article, describes good followers as follows:

   - Manage themselves well.
   - Are committed to the organization.
   - Are committed to a purpose, principle, or person outside of themselves.
   - Build their competence.
   - Focus their efforts to maximize impact.
   - Exhibit courage and honesty.
   - Achieve and sustain job-related credibility.

   Implication: Develop your ability to lead and to follow and actively develop followership skills in those who report to you.

4. *Think team, but think carefully.* A team is not a team is not a team. Hence, what leadership looks like and the appropriate focus of leaders and followers varies based on the challenge faced (e.g., the game or music played). **Robert Keidel** provides a model of this, describing the space that teams operate within as a triangular one, with autonomy, control, or collaboration at the respective angle. Teams live in different parts of the triangle at any given moment and, overall, tend to spend more time in one part of the triangle than another. This matters, again, because of the different challenges to be met or games to be played.*

   Largely autonomous teams fit challenges best described as largely individual. The "teaming" basically requires adding up the individual results. Think track and field or swim teams or recital music. The team wins if the individuals excel as individuals. The key leadership function involves se-

---

*Robert Kelley, "In Praise of Followers," *Harvard Business Review*, Nov. 1988, reprint # 88606. Robert Keidel, *Game Plans and Corporate Players* (New York: E.P. Dutton, 1985).

curing individual talent and followers need to maximize individual performance. Traditionally, most of healthcare taken as a system has operated this way and, in particular, fee for service has promoted it.

As for "control," think highly scripted and deeply interdependent. Think synchronized swimming or American football or orchestral music. A big brain leader comprises a routine or game plan or musical score and followers learn their part and adhere to it. Interdependence matters greatly— but according to the plan. Standardization of care requires playing this type of "game" although the "big brain" will have a large IT, even AI component as treatment plans and risk profiles arise from big data and dynamic programming algorithms.

Finally, "collaborative" teams play very interdependently but in largely unscripted ways. Think basketball, field hockey, lacrosse, soccer, and jazz. Team members need deep and current knowledge of their teammates in order to improvise successfully. The key leader usually lives in the fray or on the field—there's a reason that the captain of the winning team accepts soccer's World Cup. Unlike, say, American football, the coach can only infrequently stop the action. It flows and the captain has to live in the flow and influence his (or her) team's actions in real time, without a slew of time-outs and instructions from above. The captain also has to work on creating and sustaining harmony because the capacity to improvise turns on deep, spontaneous assembling of team members to deal with threat or seize opportunity. No room here for squabbling, let alone outright feuding. The part of healthcare that, by necessity, will always be art as much as science lives here, but that part should grow both more important and less common.

Implication: Figure out the game that a given group needs to play and work on leading and following accordingly.

5. *Some attributes help, except when they don't.* By and large, certain behaviors assist individuals in providing good leadership. For example, action orientation, tenacity, optimism, and participating in the work of the group. Yet, a leader who acts immediately whenever someone brings up an issue or problem may well be seen as twitchy and hence unstable and not advisable to follow. The tenacious leader who goes blind and deaf to clear warnings of failure or benefits of alternate approaches can come to be seen as simply pig-headed and not suitable to follow. The optimistic leader can deny the severity of true challenges or threats and so can come to be seen as out of touch, even detached from reality, and not suitable to follow. Finally, the leader who always joins in with the work of the team or group can come to be seen as

simply another group member, even as people begin to question who is scouting the broader environment, plotting trajectory, and obtaining resources. Hence, the appointed leader loses credibility as a leader and assigned followers come to view him or her as not suitable to follow.

Implication: Develop these four behavioral attributes, but stay current regarding your skill level and aware of your orientation, the situation, state of the team, and the needed balance Avoid the trap of holding a hammer and viewing the world as full of nails.

HOMEWORK ASSIGNMENT 3

Leading Change

Change dominates our world. It can be argued that, for most people in most organizations, their real job is change. Additionally, change as a topic let alone leading it, covers a scope of material just short of that included* under the space–time continuum. Seemingly, almost everything fits under the heading. That said, a few concepts bear highlighting for anyone setting out to lead change.

First and foremost, changing organizations in the end comes down to changing behavior. People either start doing something they did not previously do or they stop doing something that they did previously do. Absent behavioral change then, why would anyone rightly claim that change had occurred? Attitudes, motivations, and values all matter. They define our internal lives and do, indeed, guide our actions, but we determine or infer their existence by observing behavior or actions, even our own. Therefore, behavior changes or it doesn't and, accordingly, we judge that change has happened or it has not. Too much writing about change minimizes or even ignores this basic truth. Honoring it heads the change leader in a sounder and more useful direction.

The basic process that people move through in changing behavior falls roughly into three steps. The first step is *feeling a need*. Change requires energy, and for Homo sapiens, energy entails emotion. Cognitions may energize us by stirring or arousing us, but ultimately, feelings provide energy. That energy can flow from fear of a threat or from hope of achieving a de-

---

* Gregory Shea and Robert Guntner, *Your Job Survival Guide: A Manual for Thriving in Change*, FT Press, 2009.

sired end state. Fear amounts to a push ("get out of the building; there's a fire") and hope to a pull ("imagine a life filled with creative opportunities"). Fear gets people hopping quickly but drives down IQ generally and creativity particularly. Fear is also difficult to sustain. Hope opens up consideration of the possible and, given progress toward a desired end state, hope increases, but creating, sustaining, and enhancing it turns on progress, for example, through small, frequent early wins. Most change efforts draw from both sources of energy. Change leaders who can draw on different energy sources knowingly compensate accordingly, drawing more on fear, for instance, to get change moving but migrating quickly to hope for an envisioned future and developing optimism regarding its attainability.

Would-be leaders of change forget their own process through this step at their own peril. We humans can forget with remarkable ease what we move through to get to where we are. In this case, aspiring leaders of change can forget how they developed the felt need to energize their journey to change. That forgetfulness can then enable the change leaders' bewilderment and frustration (unto resentment) concerning those they would lead, those whose behavior the leader seeks to change. Such bewilderment and frustration seldom serve to aid leader–follower working relations.

The second overall step in the change process entails *envisioning alternative realities* to the one currently experienced. Restated, where do we want to go? Again, the definition of "where" could rest on fear and, in the extreme come down to "anywhere but here," or it could rest on hope and involve a specific vision of, say, "a patient-centered care operating across the continuum of a person's life" or, most likely, a mix of the two. In general, the more specific the vision, the easier to move on to the next step—namely, coming to the belief that at least one alternative to the current reality is attainable.

Specifying the alternative or the change vision assists the change leader in multiple ways. First, any would-be planner, let alone visionary, needs to move beyond what is in order to see what could be. "What is" includes both what currently exists and how one looks at it or "takes it in." Few students of perception would argue today that we take in the world as it is. **Heisenberg**, among others, established that the very act of observing changes the nature of reality. Furthermore, we bring limits, filters, and biases to our gaze. Physically, we can only see part of the spectrum of light and nothing of thermal, electromagnetic, or radiation, let alone auras—at least for most of us. Our predisposition and our capacity to "see" emotion or mood probably stems from a combination of genetic and learned "sight." So too, our experience and training heightens our ability to see parts of reality, even as it limits our ability to see others—a clinician can read signs of physical wellness and illness just as a financier can discern financial well-being (and vulnerability) and as a carpenter can quickly assess the relative healthiness of a wooden house. Our biases can even lead us to export reality in self-fulfilling ways. We can, for instance, watch for millennia as ships disappear from sight from the bottom of the hull up, indicating a curved and not a flat surface and yet, readily available data and experience notwithstanding, we as a species could conclude and contend that the Earth was flat and, therefore, forgo even considering certain travel options.

Techniques such as idealized design history of the future, backcasting, and scene creation can assist the change leader in overcoming his or her limits, filters, and biases to envision a world, a reality, a process, a service, or a product very different from what exists today. These techniques can transport a planner to another vantage point, to one freer of limits, filters, and biases of their current moment. Such transportation can free the mind to consider new possibilities or options. Additionally, these techniques can lead to discovery of an energy source for change: excitement born of envisioning a better world. Of course, joint or collaborative use of these techniques can further assist in developing the required felt need in others.*

These techniques share several attributes: They place the planner far enough out that she or he can feel freed of current constraints, and they call for creation of a detailed story to portray the working state of the future. They also rest upon the assumption that an alternative and

---

* As example, see Russel L. Ackoff, *Redesigning the Future*, New York: Wiley, 1974, and Larry Hirschhorn, *Backcasting, A Systematic Method for Creating a Picture and How to Get There*, OD Practitioner, vol. 39, n. 4, 2007, 16–21.

desired future can exist and that can be achieved. The techniques involve working backward to connect the future to the present while, again, assuming success. History of the future advocates "begin with the end in mind." Backcasting guides planners through a disciplined step-by-step backward walk from the future to the present. Working with scenes takes planners from the future to consideration of the organizational redesign necessary to yield that desired future to the changes required to produce that design.

Change leaders equipped with an elaborated desired change end state gain and what they need to move on to is step three in the change process. They acquire an enhanced ability to see just what the change will entail—namely, whose behavior and in what way. The greater elaboration also enables a more detailed analysis of what change would require and what levers of organization would need pushing (or pulling). According to the Work Systems Model, eight such levers exist: organization, workplace design, task, people, rewards, measurement, information distribution, and decision allocation. These subsystems of work organizations amount to levers of change because, in combination, they characterize an organization and produce the "at my seat" environment that drives behavior. Align the levers one way and one set of behaviors (perhaps a set indicative of little, if any, risk taking) makes sense. Align the levers another way and another set of behaviors (perhaps a set indicative of bold, if data-based, risk taking) makes sense. Ideally, change leaders would change at least half of them to drive change.

Careful consideration of the required structural change in turn helps to determine the effect on which stakeholder and in what ways. All of this analysis then helps change leaders and their potential followers to determine whether they can pull off the envisioned change that sat atop their felt need for change. The analysis also informs action planning to produce the structural changes supported by key stakeholder coalitions—both of which, in turn, increase felt need. Thus, we return to where we started: generating and maintaining felt need, the energy of change, although now, felt need flows from both the original condition or aspiration and from a far more proximate reality: work system design and the stakeholder coalitions that make that design achievable.

The Playlist

Throughout THE EVENT, our alien, wizard, time-traveling guides to the future played music that provoked and challenged. Their soundtrack caught the ear of our narrator, Steve Klasko, who has long been a Disk Jockey. When he retires, Steve will open "Stevie's Vinyl Emporium and Implantable Health Chips" on Philadelphia's South Street.

And so, here is the soundtrack for the book. Turn it up as you turn the pages, and imagine there's no blame.

THE MIX FOR THE 'MORROW OF MEDICINE

"Wasn't Born to Follow"   **The Byrds**
The competitive, autonomy, and hierarchy selection and education biases for physicians impede their chance to lead—and to follow.

"Who's Gonna Take the Blame"   **Smokey Robinson & the Miracles**
Healthcare transformation has been impeded by the fact that all the involved stakeholders have found someone else to blame.

"Time Has Come Today"   **Chambers Brothers**
Because we must create a new model for healthcare that mirrors the consumer revolution in other industries.

"More and More"   **Blood, Sweat and Tears**
An anthem to the dying fee-for-service model where doing more (not better) was rewarded regardless of outcomes.

"Let's Get Physical"   **Olivia Newton John**
Because 80 percent of a person's health is not based on doctors and drugs, but environmental factors such as nutrition and exercise.

"The Air That I Breathe"   **The Hollies**
For the same reason.

"Eat a Peach"   **Allman Brothers Band**
See "Let's Get Physical" and "The Air That I Breathe."

"With a Little Help from My Friends"   **Joe Cocker**
Because healthcare is moving to a team sport and physicians need to learn to
be part of high-powered teams.

"They Will Not Die"   **Medicine**
Because in the United States, healthcare has not dealt consistently with end-
of-life issues.

"I Feel Good"   **James Brown**
Because that's what its all about . . . access to quality healthcare and a fulfilling
healthy life.

Ten Tunes for Transformation

"Communication Breakdown"   **Led Zeppelin**
Because most readmissions occur because of the lack of communication
among hospitalists, family physicians, and the patient.

"Sorry Seems to Be the Hardest Word"   **Elton John**
Because apology is an important best practice after medical errors, despite advice physicians often receive to *decrease* communication after a mistake is made.

"Everything Has Changed"   **Taylor Swift**
What many conservatives feel since Obamacare was implemented.

"Painting Pictures"   **Adele**
Because the doctor of the future will need to develop greater observation,
creative, and communication skills.

"Changes"   **David Bowie**
2016: We will miss him. "So I turned my face to face me, but I never caught a
glimpse," because real change in healthcare occurs when we look at ourselves.

"Crossroads"   **Eric Clapton**
Because given the external access, quality, and cost pressures, health systems
are at a fork in the road and staying the same is not an option.

"Every Beat of My Heart"   **Gladys Knight & the Pips**
In honor of every hospital with a cardiovascular surgery department that
sponsors a state fair with corn dogs and funnel cakes.

"Bad Medicine"   **Bon Jovi**
In honor of an optimistic future where drug development is encouraged and drug pricing is consistent and affordable.

"(I Can't Get No) Satisfaction"   **Rolling Stones**
For all our citizens who receive inconsistent or unequal healthcare because of their race, religion, sexual orientation, or socioeconomic status.

"Wouldn't It Be Nice"   **The Beach Boys**
. . . if this book, the twelve disruptors, and the collaborative healthcare platform were real.

Interviews Unplugged

We asked 100 people to consider a "no blame" conversation about America's health care system. As you'll see in these transcripts, they were profound and moving and deeply aspirational for America's healthcare system.

They came from all the groups, whether pushing to make money, demanding to be heard, or asking to be helped. Many are major leaders of large organizations. Some are well known advocates for their communities. Others are clinicians and family caregivers. Almost all are also patients. In order to get their unvarnished ideas, we promised them anonymity. But we wrote down what they said.

We call it "Interviews Unplugged," like the MTV Unplugged music series. You hear real people without amplification talking to us.

We have printed the transcripts as a document that captures their profound thoughts about our care, our society, and the hunger for leadership. You will see the questions embedded—what's good, what's bad, what most needs to change in what you do, and what would a magic wand reveal?

WHAT'S RIGHT WITH THE AMERICAN HEALTHCARE SYSTEM TODAY

"**People** who work in healthcare go into it for all the right reasons. They care about patients." (health system leader)

"I don't believe anything's good about healthcare except that it gives people **jobs**. I know there are committed, caring, compassionate people. But there's too much wrong with it." (public health leader)

"The **resources** America has committed to healthcare and training is unparalleled. There is nothing comparable to the 141 **academic medical centers** in the United States. But for all that, we are still #17 in the world in key health indicators. We don't get value for the money we spend." (population health leader)

"Our **research** engine and the rate of innovation is remarkable. The rate of discovery and truly personalized medicine is awesome. But the way we apply that knowledge is inefficient. It's fragmented." (investor)

"A great accomplishment of our health system is **healthy aging**—the fact that people are today able to maintain a good quality of life well past the age they would have succumbed to disability or death." (community health physician)

"Doctors, nurses, and other caregivers provide **skilled, compassionate care** to appreciative patients every day. Palliative care physicians provide the most compassionate needed care. I've seen the good they do for people every day." (healthcare consultant)

"Our system does a great job at **extending life**. We are very focused as an industry at limiting preventable harm—especially after the IOM publication 'To Err Is to Be Human.' If you walk around our hospitals you will see a lot of things that make you proud because we are so focused on **safety**." (patient advocate)

"Another good thing is **compassion** of caregivers. Our technology is also incredible—I believe the finest export of the US is healthcare. You see people from all over the world come here for care. In fact, if I or a family member needed care, I would want it in the US. Probably at an urban or suburban hospital that was an academic or advanced community center." (patient advocate)

"The USA is the best place in the world to be sick, if you have insurance. Then there's **no limit** to the care that you can get, or to the level of service." (business owner)

"People think medical device companies are only in it for their profit. The reality is that most clinical research is funded by them. Without private industry, you'd get fewer advances in care. They want to make the patient better and faster." (CEO of healthcare company)

"What's best is the quality of the system for people who are extremely ill, especially for those with co-morbidities. We excel in pharmaceutical research and innovation." (leader in insurance industry)

"Little is right, but thank God there are some leading providers with at least **some ability to deal with variance and payment innovation to produce value**, such as GEISINGER (care model) and KAISER (per unit cost). It's important that they exist." (health system consultant)

"Insurance gives us the **freedom** to choose. Had a fabulous surgeon technically and humanely—engaged, accessible. Never felt lacking. Surgeon for son's surgery treated me as the caregiver." (patient)

"I had the care that enabled me to get **better faster.**" (patient)

"I had great **support** at all times." (patient)

"As a patient, I saw firsthand through my roommates that some patients in the hospital can be extremely difficult. **I commend the aides, housekeeping staff, and everyone in the hospital for the work that they do.** I have a lot of respect for them. These are tough jobs. Patients are sometimes abusive to them." (patient)

"The intentions involved in the ACA [Affordable Care Act] healthcare reforms are right. I think it is a big positive step to recognize the system is broken. Specifically, the **transparency** focus is right, the focus on quality and safety is right. The ACA rightly tries to focus on these areas, which I think are critical to achieving any kind of a functioning market for healthcare. However, the solution contained in the ACA for these areas may not necessarily be right." (health systems consultant)

"**Productivity** of physicians in the US in terms of motivation to see a lot of patients and do a lot of work is much higher than most other countries. **Michael Lewis** points out that if you rank-order countries by GDP, the characteristics for good productivity are: low taxes, . . . etc. US does very well on that score. (physician, entrepreneur)

"What we **need is optimism**. One of the great pleasures I get is thinking about my time as a practicing general internist/primary care physician and who I got to interact with. I have no regrets and have the absolute delight that **my daughter has chosen not just to be a doc but a primary care doc. That leads me to delightful chills, optimism, and excitement about the opportunities for ongoing transformation.**" (physician and health system CEO)

WHAT'S WRONG WITH THE AMERICAN HEALTHCARE SYSTEM TODAY

"**Everybody doesn't have the same access. The wealthier you are, the better care you get. There are too many excuses.**" (patient)

"Everything I wish for there are so many excuses for why it's not happening—universal care and a cure for cancer." (patient)

"If every institution in this society is at war with young black men, from schools to courts to police, why would we trust healthcare?" (community organizer)

"The machine of poverty leads to treatment of the acute care instead of helping ensure a living wage. Our social problems become health problems, and we foot the bill one way or another." (public health professional)

"**Our institutions make us unhealthy**. If a black teen male is found on the street with a drug, he goes to prison, he gets sick and abused there, and he can't have a career after that. That's about health. If a school is substandard, those children are behind for life. And make the process of reproductive health easy for women. Informed, nonjudgmental choice. It's so expensive to have a child you don't want/can't support, and sets you back." (community advocate)

"**Our healthcare, like all our politics, is about money and power**. We care less about harm. In all these areas, American policy is antithetical to health, driven by money and power: Tobacco subsidies, fast food, big trucks, and GUNS." (public health professional)

"But there is no equity in patient access even to the most fundamental of basics in healthcare. It is a bewildering system for even those that are senior execs in the system. For patients and families it is even worse."

"**The labyrinth of doom. Bureaucracy. Driven by volume we have created a medical-industrial complex that has gotten away from health and that we have to keep feeding.**" (physician and health system CEO)

"And we fail to use our patient knowledge. No other culture does end-of-life care worse than we do. It's emotionally unhealthy. We need to develop a culture that is more respectful of death and dying."

"You and I are going to live until 100. We need to think about what we can do at the age of 70 to 75 and how much we'll have to keep working to afford our healthcare." (private equity investor)

"Our system as a whole doesn't work to provide for the healthcare needs of the broader population, nor the intersection of physical and mental preventive care." (leader in insurance industry)

"We are too expensive for patients and too many people die of medical errors. I was involved in a conference where we defined medical errors the number of people that die as a result. It was suggested it could be up to 200,000 to 400,000 patients per year (equal to 10 jumbo jets crashing every week). There is not a lot of news or public outcry focused on this. One of the culprits seems to be a culture where doctors rarely share their errors and discuss them. This causes less transparency and public knowledge of this issue."

"A serious issue is communication between nurses and doctors and the hierarchy in healthcare. A friend of mine told me a story—a doctor entered a meeting late and there were no chairs and, with a hand motion, asked a nurse to get up. There is a hierarchy and sexism in the culture. This culture has gotten in the way of medical healthcare delivery." (patient and caregiver)

"Patients are too often treated as commodities—people don't remember your name, anything about you, or give you much credit for your intelligence. When my father was in the hospital, we put something on the door that said his name and his favorite sport team. We went out of our way to make people recognize him as a person."

"The whole area of healthcare is so complex and highly political, it is hard to know what to believe." (non-physician caregiver)

"It's wrong because of the way we pay for it. We got off course when we added comprehensive coverage to catastrophic coverage. As a result, there's no sense of what it costs. End-of-life is the worst example." (public health professional)

"**It's wrong because it doesn't focus on health**. People don't feel well even if their sickness is cured, if they're still overweight, smoking, and out of shape." (community advocate)

"**The ideal system would ensure that healthy people are having healthy children**. We don't do that at all. We need to ensure that today's baby grows up to have a healthy pregnancy. We need life course care. But that's not the American way—we don't do that. We don't look at all the things that keep someone healthy, from food to jobs to housing to the environment, to communities." (public health professional)

"**Sadly, the consumer is in cahoots with the medical industrial complex in what it requests**. Consumers believe that more is better. Patients almost never get that more medicine is not necessarily better medicine and that they believe that there is no downside to more medicine—cost or risk." (physician and health system CEO)

"We've made specialty surgery available to all but organized it like a factory at the expense of the patients and their families. It takes four days of PTO [paid time off] for a minor procedure: Pre-op visit, lab tests, radiology, the procedure, and follow-up. Unless you have a guaranteed job, you can't do it." (patient)

"There are so many things wrong with primary care. We could fix them, but we don't pay primary care to create integrated care—with seamless communication from doctor to lab to insurance to specialist to medical records. In fact, we undervalue and underpay primary care physicians." (*National Observer*)

"Practicing medicine has become like the financial advisor who makes money only by selling products."

"It's a for-profit business . . . the core isn't much, but the spokes are (drugs, med devices, insurance, cherry picking providers). People just don't realize how much money people make off the not-for-profit, subsidized core. Think about the millions spent on marketing where we know that our tactics in marketing healthcare have no chance to be effective but we do it for physician relations . . . for example, flyers, billboards, or print ads versus Internet search engines . . . docs complain if they don't get those things. We should spend every marketing dollar to promote healthy behaviors, not to promote individuals and promote the team with meaningless awards. We should move our marketing dollars out of physician relations." (physician)

"We need seamless technology, a team that's mine, dollars aligned around health." (patient)

"End-of-life care is mind boggling. How do we handle dementia? How do we make the last month of life the most expensive?" (religious leader)

"As we implement technology, we have too many clinicians who have learned to work around and to use the tools inefficiently. We have entire generations of providers who are not properly trained both in the utility of our systems and how to use them. We need to skate to where the puck is going to be: What is the profession of the future that we need to develop today? What are the right things to do all of the time, not just in response to the newest en vogue quality matrix?" (information technology expert)

"There is talk of developing standards of interoperability, but it is being championed by the 'losing players' as they attempt to stay relevant against large market share, closed systems.

All of the systems are based on different legacy languages, which are unable to communicate with each other. Integrating these systems for a single enterprise may encompass five or more individual programming languages. Many of these are closed systems versus open systems, which indicate their ability to link to other systems.

Hospital IT is really bad because it is boring and far from cutting edge, challenging work. We're overwhelmed by the red tape of large, cautious, conservative organizations. At the same time, payers drive a system that is not transparent and drives confusion among hospitals, providers, and patients about true value and cost." (CEO of healthcare information company)

"What's wrong is that it is simply not available for so many people. Life expectancy is going down for many groups of people in this country. We haven't done enough for folks without insurance, ethnic and racial minorities. **The disparities in health are shameful. There is still a lot of profit and racism in medicine.** We missed the boat on being more vocal in the health insurance exchanges. Now they largely serve the interests of the for-profit insurance industry. Money could have been better invested in health infrastructure—education, primary care—instead of high-tech tertiary care. We're too comfortable within our own walls—we don't go to meet people where they are. For example, our OBGYN suite looks great and has all kinds of resources and dedicated people, but pre-teen births are extremely high six blocks from here, and often those patients are getting no pre-natal care. We are not being held accountable for the health of communities." (primary care provider)

"Fee-for-service medicine and misaligned incentives impede care. It is incredible that in the United States, we have this payment system and people do not realize it is the problem. If you pay people to do things, they will do those things. Doctors are not bad people, but they are not different than lawyers, accountants, etc. **If you pay them to do more, they will do more.** The whole system is by common sense totally ridiculous. The economic reality is that fee-for-service will never work.

If you get paid to do shit, you do shit. This is just human nature." (healthcare consultant)

"Why discount care for people with insurance? Shouldn't it be the other way around? My bill had different prices for self pay versus insurance pay. **Who negotiates for people without insurance and without care?**" (wealthy patient)

"We need to continue to pursue cures and fix illness—for example, transplantation, cancer less of a death sentence, etc. We must continue to tackle Alzheimer's, cystic fibrosis, and the others. I'm glad there are people pursuing cures for things we don't know." (family caregiver)

"**I'm furious about billboards with ER waiting times on the interstate. That means you're using your ER as a profit center** because people are using it as a doctor. Hospitals are blatant about it." (patient)

"I'm having **tremendous trouble finding a primary care** doctor for my husband. His insurance changed. New recommended group: First appointment in May. They have to be full all day, but then they can't see me when I'm sick. It's getting harder and harder. Then I got a friend who knew someone to get inside and get an appointment." (family caregiver)

"There is fragmentation in healthcare system that creates tension, between payers and providers, for instance. In a fee-for-service system, providers want to increase cost of care, whereas health plans want to decrease cost. Government, meanwhile, has incentives that are not always aligned with the overall benefit of the system. Employers are pushed to manage something that they should not have to manage." (expert)

"The government is the largest employer, insurer, and policy maker; they hold a lot of the cards. The EHRs [electronic health records] are bloated because of public money. Leaders in the public sector will have to get out of the way . . . they need to do less and create the infrastructure of other market forces to do more. State licensure is a joke; doctors should be able to treat across state lines, tele-health should be reimbursed. The ACA, despite its many deficiencies was overall a step in the right direction to correct the injustice of the insurance system [denial of claims/insurance based on preexisting conditions]." (patient advocate and family caregiver)

"Most people who go into healthcare want to do the right thing—some become greedy somewhere along the way, most don't. It's a misalignment in payment system for consumers, providers, and government. Bottom line: public payers are underfunded, which causes huge cost-shifts from commercial payers and result is a hugely inefficient system."

But what's wrong is disparities in health based on race, socioeconomic status, immigration status, LGBT status, etc.

I blame the public's lack of accountability for health: no accountability for behavior. When people live unhealthy lives and get sick, they blame healthcare for being too expensive and not curing them. No one says maybe you should have lost weight, stopped smoking." (patient and family caregiver)

"We have to address end-of-life care and advanced care planning. The American healthcare crisis will not be solved until Americans accept the fact that they are going to die. The amount of money spent in the last 60 to 90 days of life in intensive care is criminal. You see futile care every day in the ICU.

I had to put a dog down one day, and I concluded **we are kinder to our pets than we are to our parents. I'm not pro–assisted suicide, but I am pro–natural death**. Patients need it to be explained that they can have a feeding tube, respirator, etc., and then die or be allowed to die. They should be given that choice." (entrepreneur and investor)

"With our country aging, if we don't dramatically improve care for aging, and demented, patients, we will have an enormous crisis. The whole concept of how to house and care for the elderly needs to be addressed, or it will bankrupt the whole nation." (national expert)

"We have to address the mental health crisis. How many ER admissions are due to mental health issues? This is a huge area of unmet need." (national lecturer on community health)

"It's unfair what we do to people at the end of life. It's almost emotional blackmail, 'what do you want to do for Uncle Johnnie?' without saying that he will be incontinent and oblivious to the world around him." (investor and entrepreneur)

"The system has moved away from a focus of the patient. Hospitals and the docs are in cahoots to produce money." (patient)

"Having an insurance-led healthcare system is a mistake. What are Americans paying for? Denmark or the Netherlands (socialist with insurance for exceptions—incredible nursing) are better models." (health system consultant)

"A health organization should bear responsibility for the health of a population and receive financial reward for providing high-quality care as close to peoples' homes as possible." (entrepreneur)

"A high-quality healthcare system should make sure patients have sufficient information to remain engaged and fully participant in their care." (insurance leader)

"Except for a handful of cases, we deliver far too much care in far too expensive settings." (specialist physician)

"We don't practice proactive and preventive health. We need to help people become committed to their own health." (chiropractor)

"My role as a stakeholder is to be the voice of the forgotten patient. Healthcare is so fragmented and difficult to understand, **we need facilitators to help and advocate** for their needs." (patient advocate)

"What's wrong? Too much of the GDP is spent on healthcare!" (patient)

"Our systems are antiquated and complicated leading to worse outcomes." (patient)

"Every aspect of the healthcare system is optimized to serve its own needs versus the needs of the patient." (patient)

"The patient has lost power. No patient engagement in preventive care." (patient)

"Finances become a health problem. It costs so much to take care of myself, and prices keep going up, that it becomes an emotional burden because I have to make choices about spending." (patient)

"What's missing: A provider/patient partnership in care." (patient)

"**Patient guilt is, at times, debilitating**. For example, I have a blood draw tomorrow, but my blood sugar went up 300, so my average is now blown, and I feel like a disappointment to the doctor and to myself." (patient)

"What's wrong is the extreme level of ignorance of our government. They don't understand the fragile nature of healthcare for vulnerable populations (elderly, uninsured, and veterans). Many hospitals don't even cover their variable costs with many elderly patients." (patient)

"Is the problem ignorance or cowardice?" (patient)

"We're trapped in a system that is designed for for-profit competition, and then the feds get into minutia to determine the matters of trade that contradict trying to develop population health." (public health practitioner)

"I'm not a fan of Obamacare, but the value statement is right. If I'm **Oliver Stone** doing this movie, Obamacare has changed the ground forever and even repealing it won't stop it. It's affected provider behavior irrevocably and for payers . . . it's now about ambulatory care & compensation . . . we need to let doomsday come faster, to adapt/reuse/close the unneeded facilities." (academic)

"Right now—we're witnessing a shameful impotence by government." (health system consultant)

"Everyone should have insurance and access to high-quality healthcare when they need it; **no one should be denied care based on their ability to pay**. We should have mechanisms in place that facilitate choice for what's rational, taking into account not only the benefits of care, but the cost and not only the effect it has on the individual, but also the effect they have on the broader polity or society. Everyone is a steward of our national resources." (healthcare policy expert)

"The inequities in our system are not compatible with a modern civilized state—with millions of Americans uninsured, people cannot afford the care that is beneficial to them even when they are insured.

We have a collective distrust of authority and concentrated power that forces us to make irrational decisions that run contrary to our own welfare. There are many problems we could solve IF we were willing to entrust more authority to some agency/organization, whether governmental or nongovernmental to allocate resources and limit what we spend in healthcare.

We have dysfunctional markets that do not reward better performance." (physician and population health expert)

"**What's wrong is Obamacare**. It has a great impact on doctors and small businesses. I have had three surgeries in the past three years and what I see are surgeons who need to double the amount of surgeries to get reimbursed the same amount as prior to Obamacare. Many small businesses are not able to provide insurance to their employees due to the cost of insurance under Obamacare." (patient)

"The intentions involved in the ACA healthcare reforms are right. I think it is a big positive step to recognize the system is broken. Specifically, the transparency focus is right, the focus on quality and safety is right. The ACA rightly tries to focus on these areas, which I think are critical to achieving any kind of a functioning market for health care. However, the solution contained in the ACA for these areas may not necessarily be right." (chief medical officer)

"Even with ACA, we have continued disparity between the actual cost of care (to the provider), the negotiated fee paid to the payer, and the cost incurred by the consumer in the form of premiums and co-pays. These three things are often so totally divorced from each other that the consumer is totally confused and doesn't understand the actual cost of healthcare. For every other industry cost is clear—there is transparency in what people are buying—there is some kind of a market-driven force. **There is so much waste in our healthcare system because of the disconnect between the actual cost of healthcare and the consumer's understanding of that cost.**" (health system consultant)

"Since I am 60 years old and my family is getting older, I have now realized that we need much better care for the elderly. Right now, I have an aunt and uncle who are older and do not have much money. They are not able to afford a nurse every day, and Medicare only provides four weeks of nursing care. Sometimes, they can't afford the prices of their medications. Medicare doesn't help with making changes to the home needed for a wheelchair. The examples are endless. These are people who worked their whole lives and Obamacare is not providing them what they need." (patient)

"We are too fast to give people with drug addictions access to Medicaid—they should be forced to go to rehab and be a productive citizen. I think we are encouraging access to Medicaid for drug addicts. I am bitter about this. It is unfair that the elderly who have worked hard all their life are not able to access or afford the care that they need, while people with drug addictions are getting healthcare at as low as 57 cents per month." (patient)

"I had wonderful care; but the payment process is corrupt. It's so large and so maze-like, almost as if designed to frustrate people. To me, there's a corruption there. *I never got a bill I could believe.*

It is morally corrupt not to be able to offer the care I got to everyone." (patient)

"Bills came up to a year later. Got dunning notice sending us to credit collector after son's surgery because insurance mistakenly categorized it as an 'accident.' It took five weeks of calls to get that bill processed by the insurance company." (patient)

"My friend with MS was forced to change doctors when employer changed insurance for cheaper rates—everything changed, meds, costs, availability." (patient)

"How do we get back that personalized care with the beauty of computerized records?" (patient)

"How do you deal with people who want to make huge profits off my pain? People who go into healthcare to make monetary profit are unethical." (patient)

"I want to see less hiding. Less collusion. Less profit making." (patient)

"As a patient I just can't make the system work. It's mind boggling to try to pull off. Even when you get to treatment, you don't know the price you're paying, and if the treatment fails, you pay again." (patient)

"Here's my list of problems:
  * Disparities of care based on differences (i.e., race, ethnicity, gender, age, sexual orientation).
  * Payment system is not aligned.
  * We don't take accountability for our health; we expect healthcare to fix us when we get sick . . . and we don't want to pay for it.
  * Misalignment among consumers, providers, and the government.
  * Medicare and Medicaid underfunded; commercial payers picking up more than their fair share.
  * Address advance care planning and deal with end-of-life issues . . . Americans don't expect to die.
  * Dramatically improve the care for the geriatric patient.
  * Address the mental health crisis in this country.
  * Regulations are way too many. A third of my time is spent on the regulatory aspects.
  * No equitable distribution of healthcare. Esp. for those that do not work." (physician entrepreneur)

"Everybody doesn't have the same access. The wealthier you are, the better care you get. There are too many excuses." (patient)

WHAT MOST NEEDS TO CHANGE

"In this perfect alien world, everyone would be an informed voter." (patient)

"Everything I wish for there are so many excuses for why it's not happening—universal care and a cure for cancer." (patient)

"I need a beautiful orchestration of mind, spirit, and body to deal with my chronic disease.

I'm grateful for the wisdom and the advances of science. But there is incomplete science: The science about how my mind works and plays into my illness is not rich enough and not recognized by my provider." (patient and patient advocate)

"Everything we are doing right now is the right thing to do in the system we operate. But this still won't work for us long term. The whole system is unsustainable.

The whole situation can be explained by this: say insurance companies take 8 percent of premiums for admin costs, 6 percent for profits, and the remaining 86 percent they actually spend on patient care. You know what they call that 86 percent actually spent on patients? They call it the medical loss ratio, and their whole business model is based on minimizing it. How can we have a working health system with this situation?" (healthcare consultant)

"Insurance companies and employers haven't had the courage to move toward value-based models. Insurers may think that value-based models make them obsolete. What we need to do is have health systems integrated into their insurance plans. This forces provision systems to make fiscally responsible decisions that benefit patients.

People say we should increase the amount of supportive care in the home, but I can't do that until I enjoy the financial rewards of keeping people in their homes. That only happens when I own my own insurance company.

A criticism of this approach is that 'consolidation is bad.' People are fearful of bigger organizations continuing on the same path of extracting greater profits from systems. But, we now have more tools to ensure quality and examples of how scale of value works. Limit my ability to extract too much profit, but do not limit my ability to gain the critical mass to effectively provide high quality care. People may react negatively to insurance companies joining forces with providers, but KAISER's hospitalization rate is HALF that of PART-NERS." (physician, [Chief Executive Officer] (CEO), and population health expert)

"We have to run the business correctly. Remove Federal Trade Commission (FTC) barriers. Identify regions: Pick the leading institutions and have them with others to manage the population and pay them based on pop health metrics. Let the analytics rule. Get the 2.6 million people or whatever you need for population health and manage them. Get the pen out and draw the lines. **A tsunami of medical need is coming our way, and they don't have nongovernmental resources. The elderly just don't and won't have the money.** We're trying to hold together a contorted system of overhead, billing complexities, and redundancy. It won't be enough. We have about one-fourth of our health system's total revenue going to Medicare loss. **Eventually, we have to have national healthcare."** (entrepreneur and venture capitalist)

"The IT problem is a subset of a much larger problem, which, if fixed, could reduce the role of government quite dramatically and quickly. In the absence of consensus on how to create a new reality for healthcare, it was necessary to put a lot of money into the IT infrastructure.

Healthcare Information Technology (IT) is about collecting and optimizing the use of the information and NOT the technology. It's not the reporting of electronic health information that is necessary, it's the use; this is where we need to invest. Organizations pursue their own self-interest; this is expected. So, there is an unwillingness of healthcare organizations to share information, and an unwillingness of vendors to facilitate healthcare information exchange. For this reason, it's going to take 10 to 20 years before we realize the benefit of information management in healthcare. I don't think that the conditions existed for successful spread of health IT when we developed 'Meaningful Use.'

People see 'Meaningful Use' as static. Stage 1 was reasonably well titrated to the capabilities of our system at the time. Some people said, "This is simple, what's the point of this?" Most physicians didn't appreciate the part where it's necessary to make your data available to patients . . . there's a public incentive. So Stage 2 of 'Meaningful Use' begins to get hard because people are not rewarded by the system for the work they need to put in. Meaningful use is viewed as a checklist." (physician insurance expert)

"Payers should share real-time information to help us adapt care rather than just wave a bit in front of us to tempt us so we'll sign with them. Payers don't share because they see it as a competitive issue. You need to be a math genius to understand each system.

We need to remember that we're all going to be patients. The patient is not at the center of today's care." (patient)

"We need a transformation—a radical change—that will yield a real market-based system that is cost effective. Problem is many people view healthcare as an entitlement, which distorts the market—if people believe they are entitled to something no matter what, it is very difficult to have a market. However, we obviously need to have a system where people can get needed care who can't afford it. But for the majority of people who are able to pay at least a portion of their care, we need to be like any other industry and have a market-based system where people know prices and are accountable for what they buy. We need a solution that forms a market-based system that holds everyone accountable. Responsibility for consumers to shop around forces the healthcare sector to become more efficient or go out of business. Market-based system like every other product or service. Also need to leave government out—too many rules and regulations that distort market. Government involvement is needed to regulate any market, but they are way too involved." (financial expert)

"Put the systems together: We need to see much more data analysis to permit new partnerships between health plans and providers. We can use the expertise in disease management residing in health plans, with the deep clinical knowledge of clinicians. We need a seamless relationship." (CEO of major insurance company)

IF YOU COULD WAVE A MAGIC WAND, WHAT ARE THREE THINGS YOU WOULD LIKE TO SAY ABOUT HEALTHCARE IN AMERICA THAT YOU CANNOT SAY TODAY?

1. **"Make healthcare a right.** Make us a system that delivers value. One that is user friendly. It will be somewhat like socialized education—like public education in the U.S.

2. We have to blow up how care delivery works. Move to a **team-based model.** Help caregivers understand new ways of taking care of people that make the

best use of resources on the team. Take the volume incentive out of the system. Put incentives in place that are aligned with the outcomes we want to have.

3. We have to confront the question of whether an employer-based system makes sense in this day and age. It may be a vestige of history. **Why should your access for healthcare be driven by who you or your spouse works for?**" (healthcare consultant)

––––––––––––

1. "The ideal system would ensure that healthy people are having healthy children. We don't do that at all. We need to ensure that **today's baby grows up to have a healthy pregnancy if she or he wishes to.**

2. We need **life course care**. But that's not the American way—we don't do that. We don't look at all the things that keep someone healthy, from food to jobs to housing to the environment, to communities.

3. Set your sights on the next generation!" (public health professional)

––––––––––––

1. "Start with the patient's role. Make them **active participants**. Data must follow patients and be structured to allow their participation.

2. Deepen understanding of communities. Most of what impacts a patient's health doesn't happen in the doctor's office. Most of what happens to the patient, happens at home. Hospitals focus on beds, their beds, not homes.

3. **Truly address access fully and completely.**" (insurance leader)

––––––––––––

1. "We need collaborative relationships in the system that benefit the patient. That's how we can create value-added care that addresses quality and cost. That means **care must be affordable.** Today, it is financially out of control.

2. That balance requires collaboration among all the participants, and I would like to see that.

3. **Most industries are transformed by people who have vision**. In the absence of that leadership, the system fails to rise. Only leadership can take the vision forward." (pharma CEO)

––––––––––––

1. "We must select students with different criteria. **We must tear up the MCAT.** We have to look for intellectual capacity and empathy. In fact, we should change all aspects of medical education.

2. The ACA reform was a good idea. Parts of it worked. We need more of it now. Focusing on population health was a good move. We need to weave it into everything we do.

3. Now it's time to talk about global capitation. The capitation initiative of the 1995 variety failed because it was on the head of the PCP. Global capitation will involve everyone. Everyone and the institution should be capitated." (population health professor)

***

1. "We should **embed healthcare education** so that it is as fundamental as reading, writing, and arithmetic.

2. Make the system work for my community. Make us the healthiest home town. Measure it against national outcomes for quality, cost, and patient satisfaction, but make it for my community. **Fight against over-doctored and over-cared for and over-charged.**

3. When I grew up, there was a sense of responsibility and service; civics and government was part of our education, which I don't see in 90 percent of the folks moving into power. Attention spans are short, jobs are transient, news is now sound-bytes. If smart people have great ideas, who is going to listen?" (entrepreneur and investor)

***

1. "Consumers will want and will see **'care in the palm of your hand.'** Consumers are far ahead of docs in the desire and willingness to use technology. This better be a wake-up call.

2. **Primary care will shift away from doctors.** There won't be a shortage.

3. That means we will have to reengineer health and medical training and schools." (finance expert)

***

1. "We need a new kind of system that is one global bucket, reliably holding active, resolved, monitored, and reported information in an intelligent manner that allows us to reliably leverage our collective knowledge for a patient. The inability to have our **information owned, managed, and shared intelligently** is a barrier that vendors need to reimagine in a way that also considers the legal implications of practitioners having potentially unlimited access to vast patient records.

2. Create an integrated system that can communicate across patient 'touch points' to allow for an **intelligent, living, health timeline for patients.** This would include past and present health problems and intelligently link

to pertinent follow-up specific to the patient while also tailoring the information so that it is specific to the provider.

3. Clinicians need to be more agile and try to understand the larger changes in healthcare outside of their scope of practice. Too many times, they have seen badly implemented and executed IS&T plans, software that doesn't work, and administrators with constantly shifting environment; find a way to just get through their day, not optimizing the product for productivity and efficiency." (physician and CEO of information technology company)

---

1. In an ideal future, we would develop an open system built with the goal of integration. **Information would be shared in a way that encourages participation of hospitals, providers, and payers in the aims of improving care and improved transparency.**

2. Only the federal government could mandate a system that would allow the leverage needed to demand a one-payer, one-system, interoperable solution—but who wants that!

3. If I had a magic wand, there would be one system or open systems, but that will never happen. No matter how high one-system market share gets, there will always be the next, newest thing right around the corner." (electronic health record expert)

---

1. "I see a world **where we get care where we are**, not where our ailment is, mostly the home and the work place. Our bodies are connected to devices that are easy to use and very inexpensive.

2. We **receive interventions in the neighborhood,** perhaps at the local pharmacy or other locations if we need to.

3. Everything is available in the cloud in a secure way, where the data that is personalized and streaming for us is being analyzed by **big data tools** that, at the end of the day, create evidence-based guidance that is much more reliable than the average physician, if you will. In that situation, we know what happened and we know what to do." (tele-health CEO)

---

1. "Why should a patient with cancer agonizing in his or her home on a snowy day have to travel to an office and get an infection that he or she doesn't deserve in a waiting room? Why should a mother with a crying baby who can't make an early appointment with her PCP have to go to the Emergency Room and get a bill that will bankrupt the family budget?

2. We should **use tele-health to embolden patients' relationships with their existing care teams.**

3. In order to effect this change, we need to **educate patients** as to how they can best be aware and engaged in these relationships." (tele-health lobbyist)

---

1. "We need more true buy-in to **restorative justice**—what led to the person being in this situation and what restitutions are available other than bail and prison. If a kid fights in school, how can we help them in a way that builds the community? Same with drugs. A kid didn't get the treatment he was supposed to get and may even have been required by law and so he acted out. **Yes, the child is responsible, but we knew what he needed and he didn't get it.** It's a mental health issue, and we pay one way or another. If 60 percent of kids in a school have trauma, then let's build a school/schooling for them.

2. We need an infrastructure and culture of health that is just like access to pharmacies and parks and schools. I stroll the same streets, but my experience is so different from that of a foster care child, for instance. She can't access WALGREEN's because foster care uses a different system. We should embed the access to resources into everyone's lives in a community. That's what we need to do to deal with the 80 percent of health that is about lifestyle. People live in families, so schools are especially important. The epicenter needs to be a quasi-public institution.

3. **Maybe the epicenter of health should be the school.** So, a kid has asthma and a physician can treat the acute event, but the child doesn't have access to chronic care and a house inspection for mold so she struggles in school and is more likely to drop out and then have a teen pregnancy, which makes her more likely to remain poor and have stress-related diseases—and we have a next generation in poverty. For males, it'd be crime. It's not just access to healthcare, it's access to health." (community advocate)

---

1. "Have a **socialist healthcare system like UK or Canada.** Our system will never work. You can look at GDP [gross domestic product] models and see the **obvious that it is doomed to collapse.**

2. We could right now do more **team-based care—integration of community health** worker, social worker, nurses, into our primary care teams.

3. The government should provide security and protection; the government should NOT become an operator. **Private-sector leaders should lead**

transformation by creating a coalition that nurtures ecosystems motivated to achieve the same goal." (healthcare consultant and primary care provider)

———

1. "Right size the industry—eliminate unnecessary **duplication**.

2. Focus more effort on **prevention**. How do we prevent people from getting sick? How do we incent healthier behaviors? How do we pay for it?

3. Align incentives among consumers, providers, payers, and government." (healthcare system consultant)

———

1. "**Tort reform**, cap on noneconomic damages.

2. **Fix the drug development** and pharma challenges of bringing drugs to market. The process of FDA [Food and Drug Administration] approval is so much more involved than anywhere else in the world. Is it safer, or has it just gone overboard? The fact there is so much unwarranted variation across the country, across markets, across hospitals is criminal.

3. **Assure equal access to preventive care**—access to care should be a universal right, but accountability for one's own health should be a universal responsibility. I would want to be able to release the following press release: 'We have eliminated all disparities of care in the American healthcare system due to race, socioeconomic status, etc.' To get there, we have to explore how we make ourselves aware of unconscious biases so we don't react in unfair ways. The American people have to **get serious about prevention**. We are what we eat. We have to start holding food companies responsible for the crap they are pushing. Why do we tolerate supersized food portions?" (health system consultant)

———

1. "I'd change the way we **drive profits through additive procedures**. For example, my 5-year-old daughter split her head. Marvelously handled. Hardly noticeable scar. The physician wanted plastic surgery and there seemed no need given her age and condition. It had to be about money.

2. I'd look at the regulations within the industry and try to figure out if the FDA is doing what it should. Look to Europe. American patients aren't getting the best medical advances as soon as they could.

3. You won't live any longer in the USA. What are we getting out of this high price for the system?" (patient/parent)

———

"I actually have four solutions for our broken healthcare system:

1. **Single-payer** system.
2. Decrease administrative expense (Medicare cards for all).
3. Encourage **integrated systems** (if can't achieve singler payer) in order to do away with insurance as it currently exists.
4. Rapidly accelerate **attraction to primary care for the best and the brightest clinicians.**" (population health expert)

---

1. "**Remove the legal and financial incentives that create overuse and over-ordering by MDs.** They're so afraid of being sued that the procedures aren't being done for the patient, they're being done for the what if.
2. A no-blame model would almost immediately improve electronic health records.
3. **Use the patient to shape physician behavior via market demand.**" (chiropractor)

---

1. "Focus resources and capabilities in a way that the patient can most easily and affordably access.
2. Use technology to its fullest potential by fully utilizing our understanding of behavioral change fundamentals to overcome perceived barriers.
3. We need to increase **patient engagement.** Let's use unique positive feedback interfaces to create a dramatic increase in **transparency** and engagement." (patient advocate)

---

1. "What would make it ideal is **if I were a valued partner.** At times, I'm left feeling like I drain time from making money with the next patient. Nothing is easy and seamless. So **nothing feels safe in the day-to-day.** There's no warm blanket of support.
2. **In a system built on trust, I would reveal more. Everything feels judgmental**—that I've done something wrong. If authentically cared about, I would reveal more of the actual struggles that exist. We fill up the time before we get to heavy things—questions about mortality and depression are easy to mask.
3. For a child with a chronic illness, we don't recognize the enormous guilt of parents. But when you have a chronic illness there is a **huge guilt of the**

patient. By revealing more, I would contribute more to my own well-being. I would be less of a burden." (patient)

---

1. "We are skirting away from our responsibility as leaders in healthcare by trying to blame our failure on others and external constraints.

2. In the future, **I dream of emotional intelligence and sensitivity being seen as the pillars of understanding.**

3. Basic process of receiving care would be easier. Why does it take an hour to find a lab? Where's the **dashboard for the patient?**" (patient advocate)

---

1. "Device innovation: Health professionals would feel **empowered by devices.** Companion sensors for sleeping, calories, movement. We have them, but they compete.

2. **We need an "EMOTION METER"** integrated into the fitness meters.

3. There is enough money in the system to provide quality care/cheaper care to all. We need to **run by analytics and be proactive.** I absolutely believe that." (entrepreneur and investor)

---

1. "We need to ensure affordability by encouraging **healthy competition within the markets of care providers to optimize quality of care,** have private-sector leaders determine the pace and means of change, and have government determine the framework within which this change occurs.

2. **We're only as healthy as our least healthy, most vulnerable segments.** We need to get back to relationships and leverage the goodness in our communities. We need to align. Otherwise we can't keep our doors open. The ignorance about healthcare is staggering.

3. Get rid of this cumbersome billing and collection. Go to one bill, one to two pages." (private equity leader)

---

1. "We must have **universal health insurance coverage.**

2. Healthcare providers/organizations should be recognized for improving quality and containing costs.

3. Reward patients for using high-quality providers and innovative models of care so that they have incentives to be a part of the solution for making healthcare more efficient and effective. If you let the market dictate func-

tionality, it won't do things that patients need, unless patients have a real voice, which they don't." (physician specialist)

———

1. "The ideal is reasonable and fair premiums, affordable drug prices, and the ability to select your provider.

2. We need a move to do away or reform Obamacare. I think **we are giving away healthcare to people who should work to be able to pay for it.**

3. All I can say is that we are capable of going to the moon and building an atomic bomb, but we cannot find a cure for cancer. It is unbelievable to me." (patient)

———

1. "America needs **cooperative politics between our parties**: if that happened, much of the rest of this might be possible. Get past political childishness. Politicians need to be polite, reach agreements.

2. In the future: **Everyone is insured!** Should be part of our normal, like Social Security, so people don't become destitute when they're ill.

3. Our system would be less fragmented where dollars aren't the primary concern. Non-profit." (patient)

———

1. "In a no-blame system, we would **eliminate unnecessary variation** in care and move to evidence-based care.

2. We would invest equally across the country in patient safety and quality initiatives.

3. We would ensure equal access to prevention and care for all who live in this country; **access to care should be a right, and accountability for your own health should be a responsibility.** In my ideal future, we have **eliminated all disparity of care** (i.e., race, ethnicity, gender, age, socioeconomic status, religion, sexual orientation) in the American healthcare system. The American people have gotten serious about preventing illness (fix the food industry; remove controllable risk factors)." (pharma executive)

Special Message to the Congress From President Harry Truman

In many ways, this remarkable message from President Harry Truman inspired the dialogue in this book. He expresses shock at the number of young people unfit for service (a percentage that is much higher today), and launches a "we can do it" appeal to Congress. But the national debate failed in 1945 and 1946 as groups campaigned against each other, sowed the seeds of distrust, and set up America's fractured constituent based healthcare system. Suppose Harry Truman had the chance to try again?

President Harry S. Truman

Special Message to the Congress Recommending a
Comprehensive Health Program

November 19, 1945
To the Congress of the United States:

As of April 1, 1945, nearly 5,000,000 male registrants between the ages of 18 and 37 had been examined and classified as unfit for military service. The number of those rejected for military service was about 30 percent of all those examined. The percentage of rejection was lower in the younger age groups, and higher in the higher age groups, reaching as high as 49 percent for registrants between the ages of 34 and 37—None of this is really new. The American people are the most insurance-minded people in the world. They will not be frightened off from health insurance because some people have misnamed it "socialized medicine."

I repeat—what I am recommending is not socialized medicine.

Socialized medicine means that all doctors work as employees of government. The American people want no such system. No such system is here proposed.

Under the plan I suggest, our people would continue to get medical and hospital services just as they do now—on the basis of their own voluntary decisions and choices. Our doctors and hospitals would continue to deal with disease with the same professional freedom as now. There would, however, be this all-important difference: whether or not patients get the services they need would not depend on how much they can afford to pay at the time.

I am in favor of the broadest possible coverage for this insurance system. I believe that all persons who work for a living and their dependents should be covered under such an insurance plan. This would include wage and salary earners, those in business for themselves, professional persons, farmers, agricultural labor, domestic employees, government employees and employees of non-profit institutions and their families.

In addition, needy persons and other groups should be covered through appropriate premiums paid for them by public agencies. Increased Federal funds should also be made available by the Congress under the public assistance programs to reimburse the States for part of such premiums, as well as for direct expenditures made by the States in paying for medical services provided by doctors, hospitals and other agencies to needy persons.

Premiums for present social insurance benefits are calculated on the first $3,000 of earnings in a year. It might be well to have all such premiums, including those for health, calculated on a somewhat higher amount such as $3,600.

A broad program of prepayment for medical care would need total amounts approximately equal to 4 percent of such earnings. The people of the United States have been spending, on the average, nearly this percentage of their incomes for sickness care. How much of the total fund should come from the insurance premiums and how much from general revenues is a matter for the Congress to decide.

The plan which I have suggested would be sufficient to pay most doctors more than the best they have received in peacetime years. The payments of the doctors' bills would be guaranteed, and the doctors would be spared the annoyance and uncertainty of collecting fees from individual patients. The same assurance would apply to hospitals, dentists and nurses for the services they render.

89. Remarks at the National Health Assembly Dinner

=

May 1, 1948

www.trumanlibrary.org/publicpapers/viewpapers.php?pid=1612

It was also my duty at that time to see that poor people were properly taken care of from a health standpoint. We had two medical men in that county at that time who devoted their whole time to the health and welfare of those people, who couldn't afford to pay for medical care. We had an excellent county home which had a population on the average of about eight hundred all the time. And Kansas City had a hospital which contained from five to seven hundred, all the time, of people who could not afford medical care in any other way. They were indigent. And I found out with that experience that the people at the indigent bottom of the scale and the people at the top of the scale were the only ones who can afford adequate hospital care and medical care. And I became vitally interested in that situation. . . .

You know, the most of us, the reason we are not physically fit is because we are too lazy to take care of ourselves. We sit down and wait until this paunch comes on, and when we get bent over, then we try to correct it by heroic methods; and 9 times out of 10, if you go along and do what you ought to, in the first place, you wouldn't have that situation.

List of Acronyms

ACOs	accountable care organizations
API	application program interface
AI	augmented intelligence
BNB	"Blackout to No Blame" or Believe, not Blame (BNB)
CASTLS	Centers for Assessment of Surgical and Teamwork Learning and Simulation
CGs	(cool geeks)
CHIMPS	changes in mandatory programs
CEO	chief executive officer
CIO	chief information officer
D-5	Disruptive Dozen Dimensions of a Dramatically Different Healthcare for America
DDDD	Dramatically Different Democratic Discourse
EBITA	earnings before interest, taxes, and amortization
EHR	electronic health record
EMR	electronic medical records
f2f	face-to-face
FMEA	failure mode and effects analysis
FDA	Food and Drug Administration
HRO	high-reliability organization
IFTTT	If This Then That
IS&T	information systems and technology
IT	information technology
IOM	Institute of Medicine
IRB	institutional review board
IoT	Internet of Things
ISPs	Internet service providers

RRRRR	Let's Re-imagine a Republican Revolution in Healthcare, Rather Than Repeal MCAT
MWGC	Milky Way Galaxy Centric
NIH	National Institutes of Health
OMG	On My Game
OECD	Organization for Economic Cooperation and Development
PCMH	patient-centered medical home
PWI	Personal Well-Being Implant
SHADES	super hi-def analytic decision engine systems
UFO	unusually frank and open
USNIR	*US News and Interplanetary Report*
USNWR	*US News and World Report*

Index

Note: footnote information is denoted with an n following the page number.